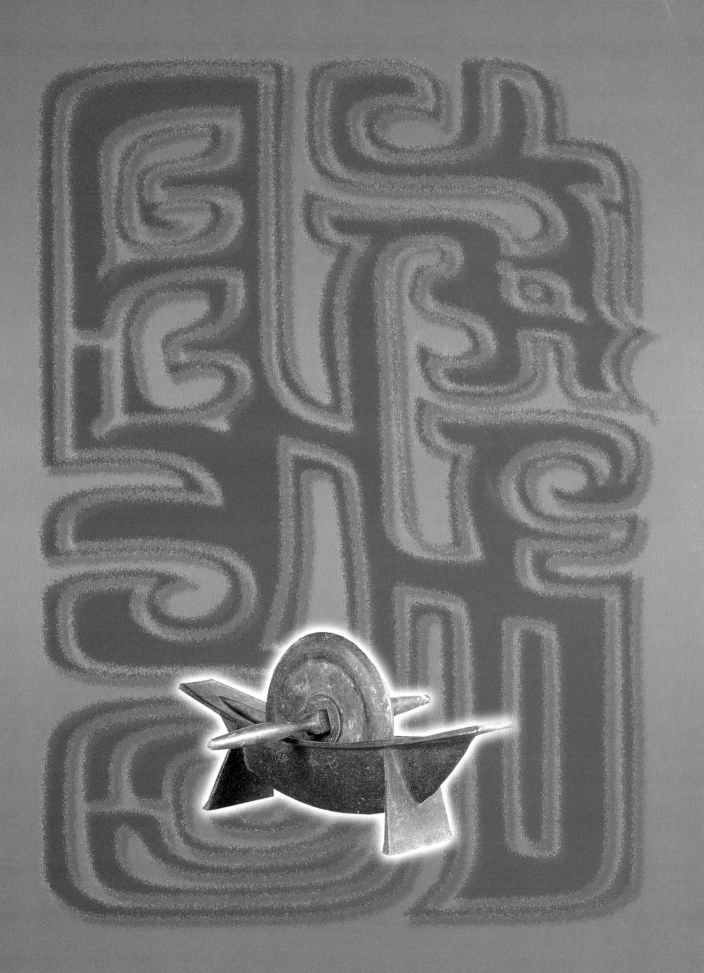

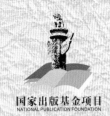

国家出版基金项目
NATIONAL PUBLICATION FOUNDATION

中华医药卫生

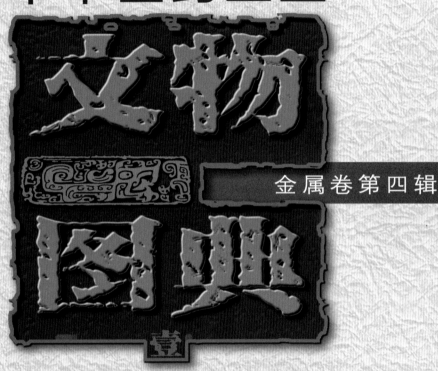

金属卷第四辑

主　编　李经纬　梁　峻　刘学春
总主译　白永权
主　译　范晓晖　郭　梦

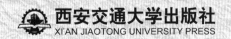

西安交通大学出版社
XI'AN JIAOTONG UNIVERSITY PRESS

图书在版编目 (CIP) 数据

中华医药卫生文物图典 . 1. 金属卷 . 第 4 辑 . / 李经纬，
梁峻，刘学春主编 . — 西安：西安交通大学出版社，2016.12

ISBN 978-7-5605-7026-6

Ⅰ . ①中… Ⅱ . ①李… ②梁… ③刘… Ⅲ . ①中国医药学 —
金属器物 — 古器物 — 中国 — 图录 Ⅳ . ① R-092 ② K870.2

中国版本图书馆 CIP 数据核字（2015）第 022428 号

书　　名	中华医药卫生文物图典（一）金属卷第四辑	
主　　编	李经纬　梁　峻　刘学春	
责任编辑	张沛烨	

出版发行　西安交通大学出版社

　　　　　（西安市兴庆南路 10 号　邮政编码 710049）

网　　址　http://www.xjtupress.com

电　　话　（029）82668805　82668502（医学分社）

　　　　　（029）82668315（总编办）

传　　真　（029）82668280

印　　刷　中煤地西安地图制印有限公司

开　　本　889mm×1194mm　1/16　印张 35.5　字数 555 千字

版次印次　2017 年 12 月第 1 版　2017 年 12 月第 1 次印刷

书　　号　ISBN 978-7-5605-7026-6

定　　价　980.00 元

读者购书、书店添货、如发现印装质量问题，请通过以下方式联系、调换。

订购热线：（029）82665248　（029）82665249

投稿热线：（029）82668805　（029）82668502

读者信箱：medpress@126.com

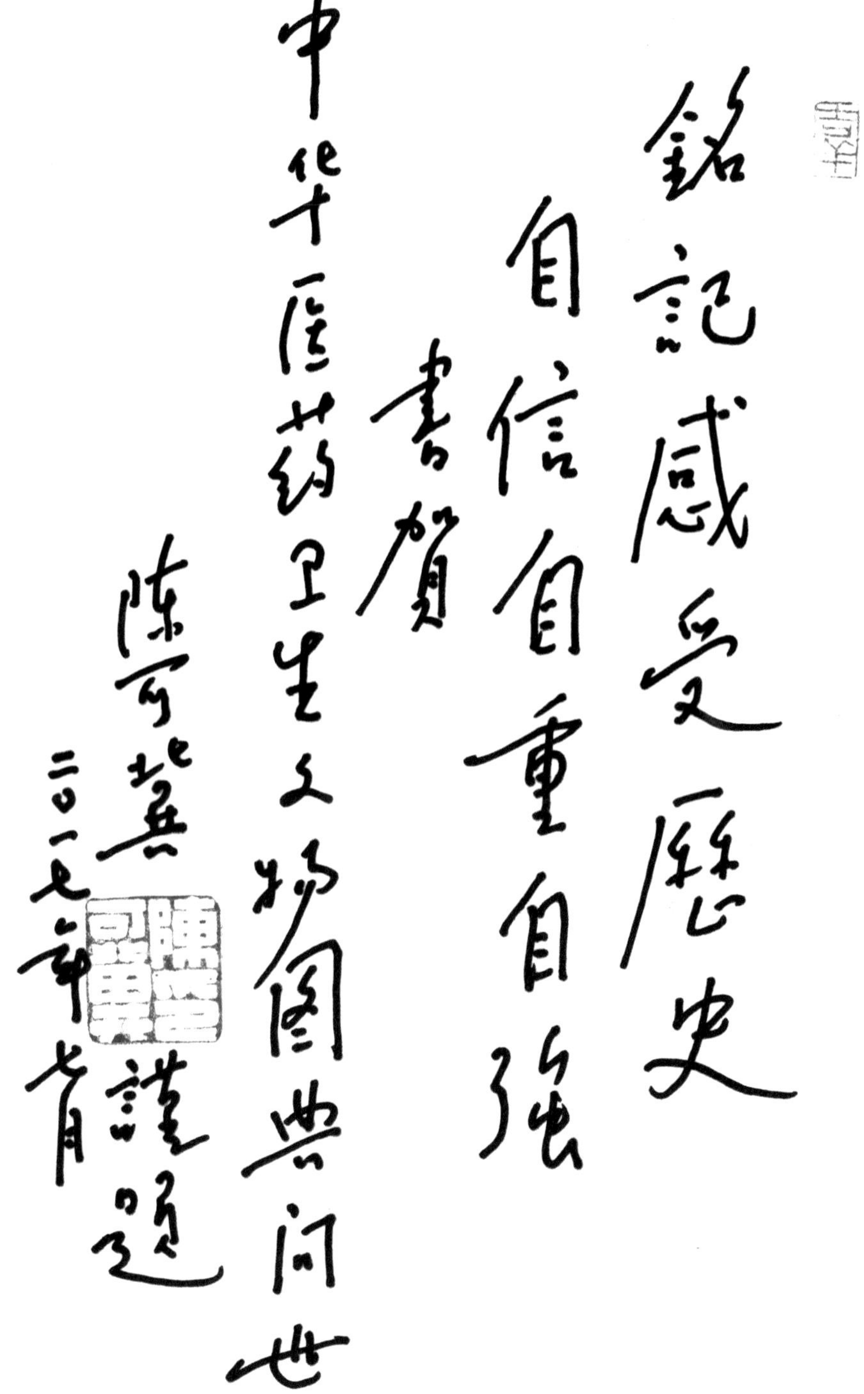

铭记感受历史

自信自重自强

书贺

中华医药卫生文物图典问世

陈可冀 谨题

二〇一七年春月

陈可冀　中国科学院院士、国医大师

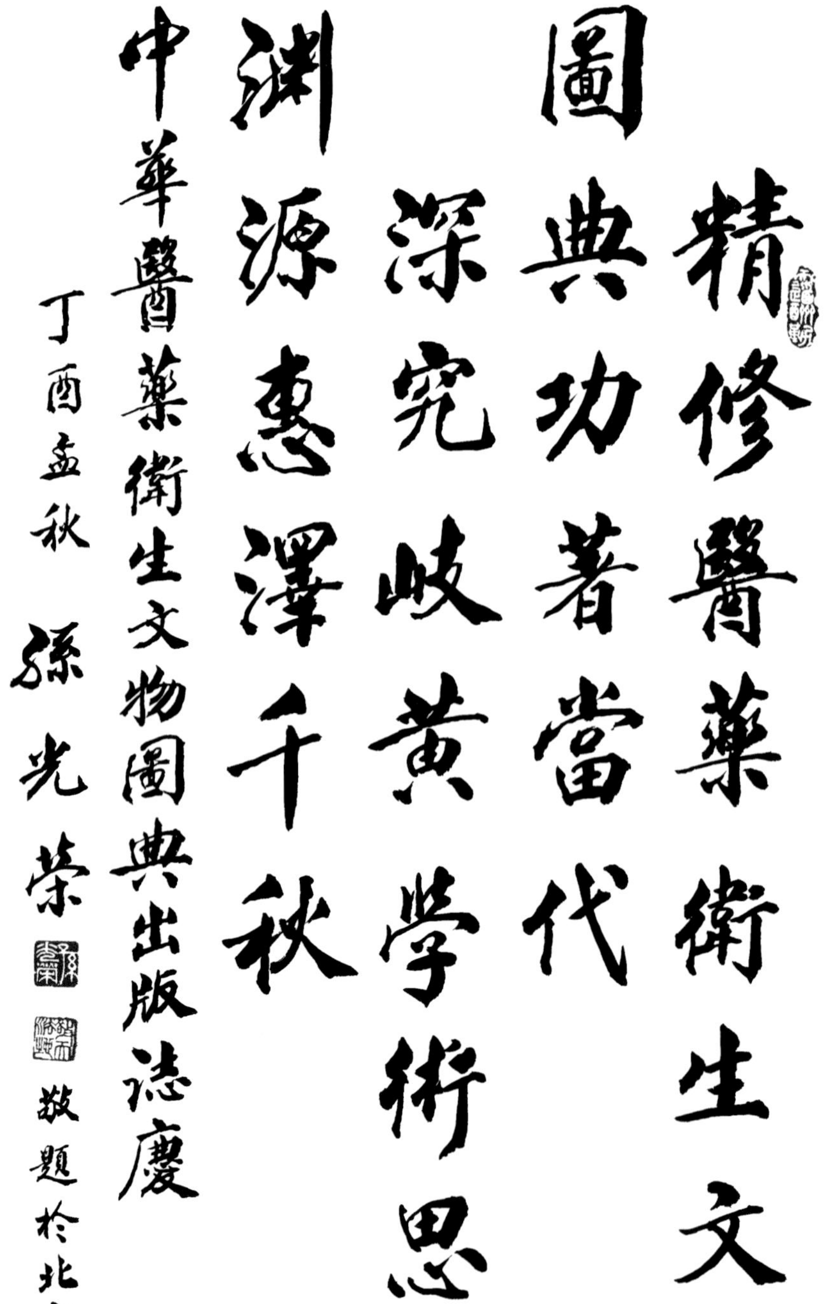

精修醫藥衛生文物

圖典功著當代

深究岐黃學術思想

淵源惠澤千秋

中華醫藥衛生文物圖典出版誌慶

丁酉孟秋 孫光榮 敬題於北京

孙光荣　国医大师

中華醫藥 衛生文物圖典出版

彰顯中醫藥
文化精神

體現中醫藥
歷史價值

歲次丁酉夏　王琦

王琦　国医大师

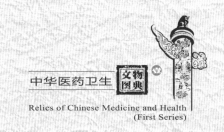

中华医药卫生

Relics of Chinese Medicine and Health
(First Series)

中华医药卫生文物图典（一）
丛书编撰委员会

主　编　李经纬　梁　峻　刘学春

副主编　廖　果　吴鸿洲　康兴军　和中浚　刘小斌　杨金生

　　　　　郑怀林　徐江雁　白建疆　黄　煌

编　委　李洪晓　梁永宣　王强虎　董树平　马　健　王　霞

　　　　　张雅宗　朱德明　包哈申　张建青　郑　蓉　庄乾竹

　　　　　李宏红　刘哲峰　王宏才　陈润东

总主译　白永权

主　译　陈向京　聂文信　范晓晖　温　睿　赵永生　杜彦龙

　　　　　吉　乐　李小棉　郭　梦　陈　曦

副主译（按姓氏音序排列）

　　　　　董艳云　姜雨孜　李建西　刘　慧　马　健　任宝磊

　　　　　任　萌　任　莹　王　颇　习通源　谢皖吉　徐素云

　　　　　许崇钰　许　梅　詹菊红　赵　菲　邹郝晶

译　者（按姓氏音序排列）

迟征宇　邓　甜　付一豪　高　琛　高　媛　郭　宁

韩　蕾　何宗昌　胡勇强　黄　鋆　蒋新蕾　康晓薇

李静波　刘雅恬　刘妍萌　鲁显生　马　月　牛笑语

唐云鹏　唐臻娜　田　多　铁红玲　佟健一　王　晨

王　丹　王　栋　王　丽　王　媛　王慧敏　王梦杰

王仙先　吴耀均　席　慧　肖国强　许子洋　闫红贤

杨姣姣　姚　晔　张　阳　张　鋆　张继飞　张梦原

张晓谦　赵　欣　赵亚力　郑　青　郑艳华　朱江嵩

朱瑛培

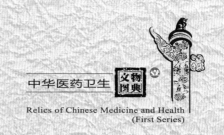

Relics of Chinese Medicine and Health
(First Series)

本册编撰委员会

主　编　李经纬　梁　峻　刘学春

副主编　廖　果　吴鸿洲　康兴军　和中浚　刘小斌　杨金生

　　　　郑怀林　徐江雁　白建疆　黄　煌

编　委　李洪晓　梁永宣　王强虎　董树平　马　健　王　霞

　　　　张雅宗　朱德明　包哈申　张建青　郑　蓉　庄乾竹

　　　　李宏红　刘哲峰　王宏才　陈润东

总主译　白永权

主　译　范晓晖　郭　梦

副主译　李建西　任宝磊

译　者　闫红贤　赵　欣　朱江嵩　赵亚力　马　月　赵　菲

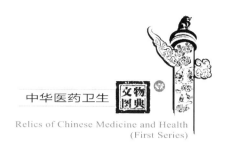

中华医药卫生 文物图典

Relics of Chinese Medicine and Health
(First Series)

序 言

探索天、地、人运动变化规律以及"气化物生"过程的相互关系，是人类永恒的课题。宇宙不可逆，地球不可逆，人生不可逆业已成为共识。天地造化形成自然，人类活动构成文化。文物既是文化的载体，又是物化的历史，还是文明的见证。

追求健康长寿是人类共同的夙愿。中华民族之所以繁衍昌盛，健康文化起了巨大的推动作用。由于古人谋求生存发展、应对环境变化产生的智慧，大多反映在以医药卫生为核心的健康文化之中，所以，习总书记说："中医药学是中国古代科学的瑰宝，也是打开中华文明宝库的钥匙"。

秉持文化大发展、大繁荣理念，中国中医科学院李经纬、梁峻等为负责人的科研团队在完成科技部"国家重点医药卫生文物收集调研和保护"课题获 2005 年度中华中医药学会科技二等奖基础上，又资鉴"夏商周断代工程""中华文明探源工程"等相关考古成果，用有重要价值的新出土文物置换原拍摄质量较差的文物，适当补充民族医药文物，共精选收载 5000 余件。经西安交通大学出版社申报，《中华医药卫生文物图典（一）》（以下简称《图典》）于 2013 年获得了国家出版基金的资助，并经专业翻译团队翻译，使《图典》得以面世。

文物承载的信息多元丰富，发掘解读其中蕴藏的智慧并非易事。医药卫生文物更具有特殊性，除文物的一般属性外，还承载着传统医学发展史迹与促进健康的信息。运用历史唯物主义观察发掘文物信息，善于从生活文物中领悟卫生信息，才能准确解读其功能，也才能诠释其在民生健康中的历史作用，收到以古鉴今之效果。"历史是现实的根源"，任何一个民族都不能割断历史，史料都包含在文化中。"文化是民族的血脉，是人民的精神家园"，文化繁荣才能实现中华民族的伟大复兴。值本《图典》付梓之际，用"梳理文化之脉，必获健康之果"作为序言并和作者、读者共勉！

中央文史研究馆馆员
中国工程院院士　　王永炎
丁酉年仲夏

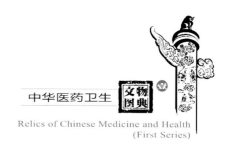

中华医药卫生 文物图典

Relics of Chinese Medicine and Health
(First Series)

前 言

　　文化是相对自然的概念，是考古界常用词汇。文物是文化的重要组成部分，既是文明的物证，又是物化的历史。狭义医药卫生文物是疾病防治模式语境下的解读，而广义医药卫生文物则是躯体、心态、环境适应三维健康模式下的诠释。中华民族是 56 个民族组成的多元一体大家庭，中华医药卫生文物当然包括各民族的健康文化遗存。

　　天地造化如造山、板块漂移、气候变迁、生物起源进化等形成自然。气化物生莫贵于人，即整个生物进化的最高成果是人类自身。广义而言，人类生存思维留下的痕迹即物质财富和精神财富总和构成文化，其一般的物化形式是视觉感知的文物、文献、胜迹等。其中质变标志明晰的文化如文字、文物、城市、礼仪等可称作文明。从唯物史观视角观察，狭义文化即精神财富，尤其体现人类精、气、神状态的事项，其本质也具有特殊物质属性，如量子也具有波粒二相性，这种粒子也是物质，无非运动方式特殊而已。现代所谓可重复验证的"科学"，事实上也是从文化中分离出来的事项，因此也是一种特殊文化形式。追求健康长寿是人类共同的夙愿。中华民族之所以繁衍昌盛，是因为健康文化异彩纷呈。中华优秀传统医药文化之所以博大精深，是因为其原创思维博大、格物致知精深，所以，习总书记说："中医药学是中国古代科学的瑰宝，也是打开中华文明宝库的钥匙"。

文化既反映时代、地域、民族分布、生产资料来源、技术水平等信息，又反映人类认知水平和生存智慧。发掘解读文物、文献中蕴藏的健康知识和灵动智慧，首先是从事健康工作者的责任和义务。《易经》设有"观"卦，人类作为观察者，不仅要积极收藏展陈文物，而且要善于捕捉文物倾诉的信息，汲取养分，启迪思维，收到古为今用之效果。墨子三表法，首先一表即"本之于古者圣王之事"，也是强调古代史实的重要性。"历史是现实的根源"，现实是未来的基础。任何一个国家、地区、民族都不能割断历史、忽略基础，这个基础就是文化。"文化是民族的血脉，是人民的精神家园"。文化繁荣才能驱动各项事业发展，才能实现中华民族的伟大复兴。

人类从类人猿分化出来。"禄丰古猿禄丰种"是云南禄丰发现的类人猿化石，距今七八百万年。距今200万年前人类进入旧石器时代，直立行走，打制石器产生工具意识，管理火种，是所谓"燧人氏"时代。中国留存有更新世早、中期的元谋、蓝田、北京人等遗址。距今10万—5万年前，人类进入旧石器时代中期，即早期智人阶段，脑容量增加，和欧洲、非洲人种相比，原始蒙古人种颧骨前突等，是所谓"伏羲氏"时代。中国发现的马坝、长阳、丁村人等较典型。距今5万—1万年前，人类进入旧石器时代晚期，即晚期智人阶段，细石器、骨角器等遍布全国，山顶洞、柳江、资阳人等较典型。

中石器时代距今约1万年，是旧石器时代向新石器时代的短暂过渡期，弓箭发明，狗被驯化。河南灵井、陕西沙苑遗址等作为代表。距今1万—公元前2600年前后，人类进入新石器时代，磨光石器、烧制陶器，出现农业村落并饲养家畜，是所谓"神农氏"时代。公元前7000年以来，在甲、骨、陶、石等载体上出现契刻符号、七音阶骨笛乐器等，反映出人文气息趋浓。公元前6000—公元前3500年的老官台、裴李岗、河姆渡、马家浜、仰韶等文化遗址，彰显出先民围绕生存健康问题所做的各种努力。

公元前4800年以来，以关中、晋南、豫西为中心形成的仰韶文化，是中原史前文化的重要标志。以半坡、庙底沟类型为典型，自公元前3500年走向繁荣，属于锄耕粟黍稻兼营渔猎饲养猪鸡经济方式，彩陶尤其发达。公元前4400—公元前3300年，长江中游的大溪文化，薄胎彩陶和白陶发达。公元前4300—公元前2500年山东丰岛的大汶口文化，红陶为主。公元前3500年前后，辽东的红山文化原始宗教发展。公元前3300年以来，长江下游由河姆渡、马家浜文化衍续的良渚文化和陇西的马家窑文化、江淮间的薛家岗文化时趋发达。

公元前2600—公元前2000年，黄河中下游龙山文化群形成，冶铸铜器，制作玉器，土坯、石灰、夯筑技术开始应用。公元前2697年，轩辕战败炎帝（有说其后裔）、蚩尤而为黄帝纪元元年。黄帝西巡访贤，"至岐见岐伯，引载而归，访于治道"。其引归地"溱洧襟带于前，梅泰环拱于后"，即今河南新密市古城寨。岐黄答问，构建《黄帝内经》健康知识体系，中华文明从关注民生健康起步。颛顼改革宗教，神职人员出现；帝喾修身节用，帝尧和合百国，舜同律度量衡，大禹疏导治水，中华民族不断繁衍昌盛。

公元前2070年，禹之子启以豫西晋南为中心建立夏王朝，二里头青铜文化为其特征，半地穴、窑洞、地面建筑并存。饮食卫生器具、酒器增多。朱砂安神作用在宫殿应用。公元前1600年，商灭夏。偃师商城设有铸铜作坊。公元前1300年，盘庚迁殷，使用甲骨文。武丁时期青铜浑铸、分铸并存。公元前1056年，相传周"文王被殷纣拘于姜里，演《周易》，成六十四卦"。公元前1046年，武王克商建周，定都镐京。青铜器始铸长篇铭文，周原发掘出微型甲骨文字。公元前770年，平王东迁。虢国铸铜柄铁剑。公元前753年，秦国设置史官。公元前707年出现蝗灾、公元前613年出现"哈雷彗星"，均被孔子载入《春秋》。公元前221年，秦始皇统一中国，多元一体民族大家庭形成，中华医药卫生文物异彩纷呈。

中国是治史大国，历来重视发展文化博物事业，1955年成立卫生部中医研究院时就设置医史研究室，1982年中国医史文献研究所成立时复建中国医史博物馆研究收藏展陈文物。2000—2003年，经王永炎院士、姚乃礼院长等呼吁，科技部批准立项，由李经纬、梁峻为负责人的团队完成"国家重点医药卫生文物收集调研和保护"项目任务，受到科技部项目验收组专家的高度评价，获中华中医药学会科技进步二等奖。2013年，在国家出版基金资助下，课题组对部分文物重新拍摄或必要置换、充实民族医药文物后，由西安交通大学出版社编辑、组聘国内一流翻译团队英译说明文字付梓，受到国家中医药博物馆筹备工作领导小组和办公室的高度重视。

"物以类聚"，《图典》主要依据文物质地、种类分为9卷，计有陶瓷，金属，纸质，竹木，玉石、织品及标本，壁画石刻及遗址，少数民族文物，其他，备考等卷。同卷下主要根据历史年代或小类分册设章。每卷下的历史时段不求统一。遵循上述规则将《图典》划分为 21 册，总计收载文物 5000 余件。对每件文物的描述，除质地、规格、馆藏等基本要素外，重点描述其在民生健康中的作用。对少数暂不明确的事项在括号中注明待考。对引自各博物馆的材料除在文物后列出馆藏外，还在书后再次统一列出馆名或参考书目，以充分尊重其馆藏权，也同时维护本典作者的引用权。

21 世纪，围绕人类健康的生命科学将飞速发展，但科学离不开文化，文化离不开文物。发掘文物承载的信息为现实服务，谨引用横渠先生四言之两语："为天地立心，为生民立命"，既作为编撰本《图典》之宗旨，也是我们践行国家"一带一路"倡议的具体努力。希冀通过本《图典》的出版发行，教育国人，提振中华民族精神；走向世界，为人类健康事业贡献力量。

李经纬　梁峻　刘学春

2017 年 6 月于北京

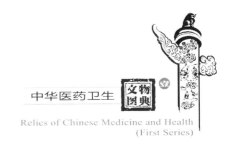

中华医药卫生文物图典

Relics of Chinese Medicine and Health
(First Series)

目 录

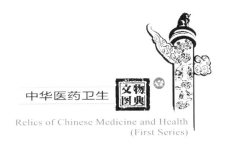

中华医药卫生 文物图典

Relics of Chinese Medicine and Health
(First Series)

contents

Chapter Three   Liao, Song, Jin, and Yuan Dynasties

◇ 第一章　魏晋南北朝

Chapter One　Wei, Jin, Southern and Northern Dynasties

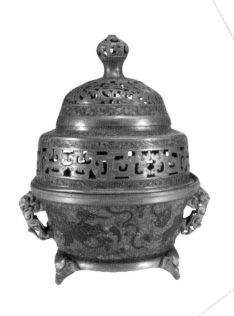

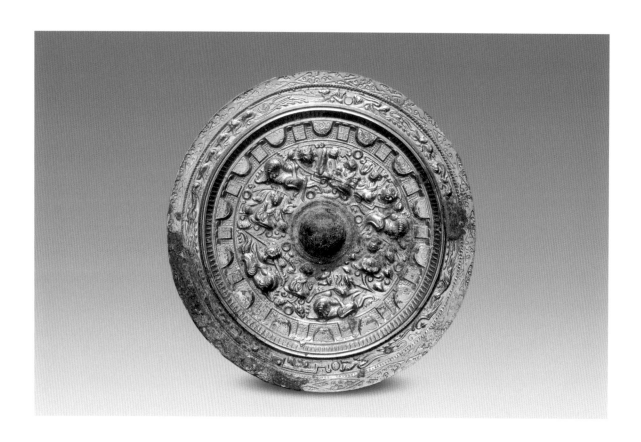

神兽镜

三国·魏

铜质

直径 15 厘米

Mirror with Supernatural Figures and Animals

Wei State, Three Kingdoms

Bronze

Diameter 15 cm

圆形。圆钮，卷草纹钮座。主纹饰分为三段，上段人像三尊，坐一长条案台上，台两侧各饰一兽。中间一人为伯牙弹琴。中段左侧一人坐于二兽座上，右侧一人坐于莲花座上，应是东王公、西王母。下段一人端坐于台上，应是黄帝。台两侧饰龙虎纹。外为菱形纹，菱形内饰卷草纹。河南省洛阳市出土。

中国国家博物馆藏

The mirror is circular in shape and has a hemispherical knob on a knob base decorated with scroll patterns. The main pattern consists of three segments. In the upper segment there are three figures sitting at a table with two animals at each end. The person in the middle is Boya, who is playing the Qin, an ancient musical instrument. The two figures in the middle segment are the King of the East, who is sitting on two animals on the left side, and the Queen of the West, who is sitting on a lotus base on the right side. The figure in the lower segment is the Emperor who is sitting on a base decorated with dragon and tiger patterns on both sides. The exterior ring has diamond-shaped patterns with scroll patterns in each diamond. The mirror was unearthed in Luoyang City, Henan Province.

Preserved in National Museum of China

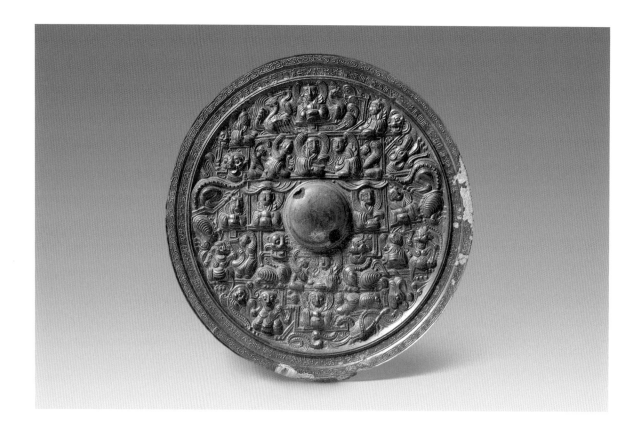

硕人神兽镜

三国·吴

铜质

直径 14.8 厘米

Mirror with Supernatural Figures and Animals

Wu State, Three Kingdoms

Bronze

Diameter 14.8 cm

圆形。圆钮，圆形钮座。纹饰横列成五排。第一排中间坐一神人，两边是神鸟神兽和侧坐神人。第二排中间置一神人，侧旁各有两人舞蹈，其外为神兽。第三排钮两侧各坐两神人，外侧各有一神兽。第四排中间饰神人，两侧为神人神兽。第五排中间坐一神人，两边饰神兽。镜缘处有铭文一周，八十八字，为《诗经·卫风·硕人》篇。此镜铸作精美，以《诗经》入镜，颇为少见。1970年湖北省武汉市征集。

武汉市文物商店藏

This circular mirror has a hemispherical knob with a circular knob base. The patterns on its back are arranged in five rows. There is an immortal being sitting in the middle of the first row with supernatural birds, animals and other supernatural beings on his both sides. In the next row there is also an immortal being in the middle with two figures dancing around him and mythical animals even farther. In the middle of the third row there is a knob with two supernatural beings sitting on each side and one mythical animal even farther. In both the fourth and fifth rows there is an immortal being in the middle respectively. The one in the fourth row has supernatural beings and animals on his both sides while the one in the fifth row has only supernatural animals on his sides. An 88-word poem from *the Book of Songs* is inscribed on the edge of the mirror. The mirror was cast with such exquisite workmanship and had *the Book of Songs* incorporated in it, which is very rare. The mirror was collected in Wuhan City, Hubei Province, in 1970.

Preserved in Wuhan Antique Store

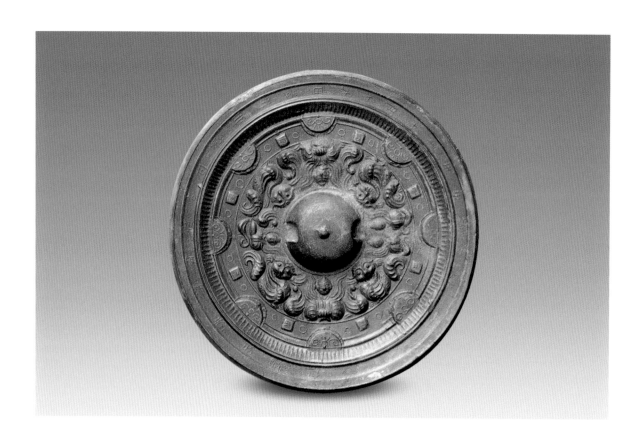

永安五年神兽镜

三国·吴

铜质

直径 12.1 厘米

Supernatural Animal Mirror of the Fifth Year of Yong`an Period

Wu State, Three Kingdoms

Bronze

Diameter 12.1 cm

圆形。圆钮，钮平，顶上有一小钉，圆钮座。钮外
四组神人与四兽相间配列，其中钮上、下两组神人
左右各一昂首翘尾鸾鸟，钮左神人身左侧立一鸾鸟，
钮右两神人对坐。外围有圆弧、方枚各八相间环绕
一周。圆弧上饰勾连云纹，方枚上各铸一字，字迹
不清。外有栉纹带一周，周外有铭文二十七字。

中国国家博物馆藏

The circular mirror has a hemispherical knob. There
is a small nipple on the flat top of the knob, the base
of which is circular. Four sets of motifs are distributed
alternately around the knob. The sets above and
underneath the knob are supernatural beings with a
bird holding its head and tail high on each side. On the
left side of the knob is a supernatural being with a bird
on his left. The other two supernatural beings sitting
opposite to each other are on the right side of the knob.
Outside the four sets are eight squares interspersed
with eight semicircles decorated with interlocking
cloud patterns. There are faded inscriptions cast in the
eight squares. A circle of comb patterns enclose all the
other motifs. Twenty-seven words are inscribed on the
edge of the mirror.

Preserved in National Museum of China

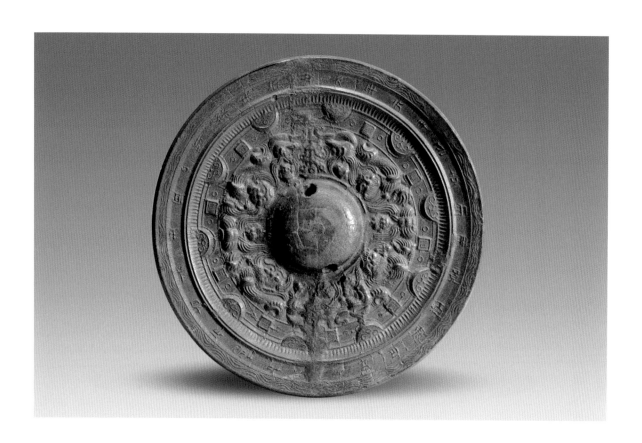

太平元年神兽镜

三国·吴

铜质

直径 14.5 厘米

Supernatural Animal Mirror of the First Year of Taiping

Wu State, Three Kingdoms

Bronze

Diameter 14.5 cm

圆形。圆钮，圆钮座。座外高浮雕神兽纹及半圆方枚相间，纹饰呈环绕式排列。镜边一圈铭文，有"太平元年"（256）的纪年。其外饰一周水波纹。1977年安徽省肥西县出土。

安徽博物院藏

The mirror itself, its knob, and the knob base are all circular. Distributed around the knob base in high relief are supernatural animals surrounded by squares and semicircles arranged alternately on the outside. The edge of the mirror is inscribed with the Chinese characters "Tai Ping Yuan Nian", meaning that the mirror was made in the first year of Taiping (256). The characters are surrounded by a circle of wave patterns. The mirror was unearthed in Feixi County, Anhui Province, in 1977.

Preserved in Anhui Museum

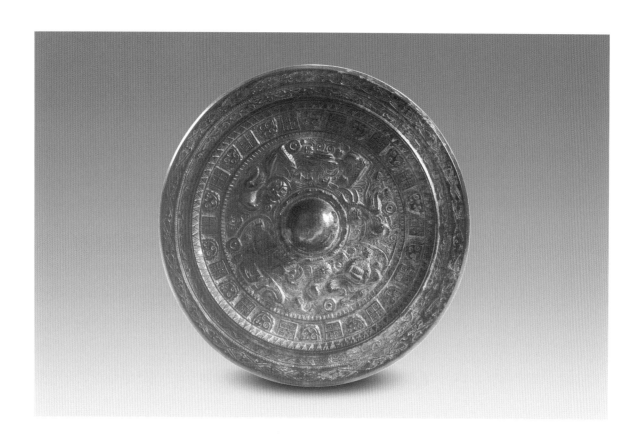

泰始九年神兽镜

西晋（泰始九年，273 年）

铜质

直径 17.6 厘米，缘厚 0.6 厘米

Supernatural Animal Mirror of the Ninth Year of Taishi

Western Jin Dynasty（The Ninth Year of Taishi, 273）

Bronze

Diameter 17.6 cm/ Rim Thickness 0.6 cm

圆形。圆钮，连珠纹钮座。镜面微弧，镜背下凹，镜背纹饰以锯齿纹为界分为两区，内区饰高浮雕人物、神兽及四枚环状乳；外区饰半圆方形带，有钤印式铭文："泰始九年 三月七日 张氏作青 同（铜）竟（镜）□大 工青且明 泰九年作 明如日月 光上有东 王父泰□ 西王母□ 食□天生 如金石位 至三公世 世公侯王" 每印四字，计64字。镜缘内亦饰锯齿纹，缘上饰画纹带。1983年河南省淇县出土。

河南博物院藏

This circular mirror has a circular knob and the knob base is decorated with a ring of pearl patterns. The mirror has a slightly curved surface and its back is concave. The motifs on its back are divided into two segments by a ring of dented patterns. In the inner segment there are figures, supernatural animals and four nipples in high relief, while in the outer segment there is a circle of semicircles and squares, the latter containing 64 inscriptions. The inner rim of the mirror is also decorated with dented patterns. On the rim there is a circle of decorative patterns. The mirror was unearthed in Qi County, Henan Province, in 1983. Preserved in Henan Museum

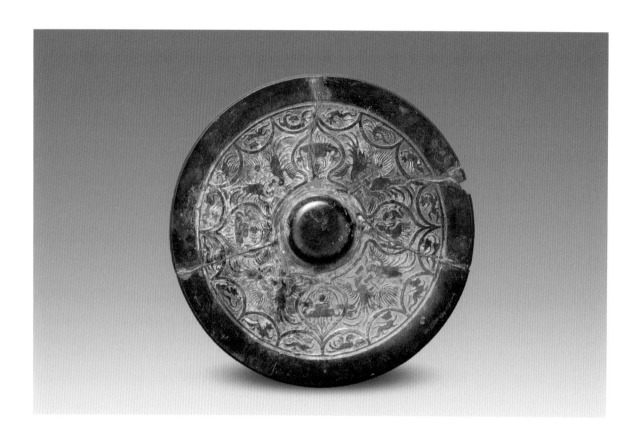

八凤佛像镜

西晋

铜质

直径 16.3 厘米

Mirror of Eight Phoenixes and Buddha

Western Jin Dynasty

Bronze

Diameter 16.3 cm

圆形。圆钮，圆钮座，宽平缘。主纹为四桃

形叶与展翅翘尾的对凤，四叶瓣内有佛像，

其中三叶内各饰一尊坐像，端坐于龙首莲花

座上。另一叶内饰像三尊，主尊居中，侧坐

于莲花座上，两侧为侍者，一跪一立。边缘

为十六连弧纹，弧内饰龙、虎、飞鸟、奔兽等。

1975 年湖北省鄂州市鄂城区出土。

中国国家博物馆藏

The mirror is circular with a wide and flat rim. Its knob and knob base are both circular. The principal motifs are four sets of paired flying phoenixes interspersed with four heart-shaped leaves. One Buddha figure is sitting on a lotus base in each of three leaves. On the fourth leaf there are three Buddha figures, the principal one sitting in the middle with one attendant on each side. The edge is decorated with sixteen continuous arc patterns combined with dragons, tigers, birds and running animals. The mirror was unearthed in Echeng District of Ezhou City, Hubei Province, in 1975.

Preserved in National Museum of China

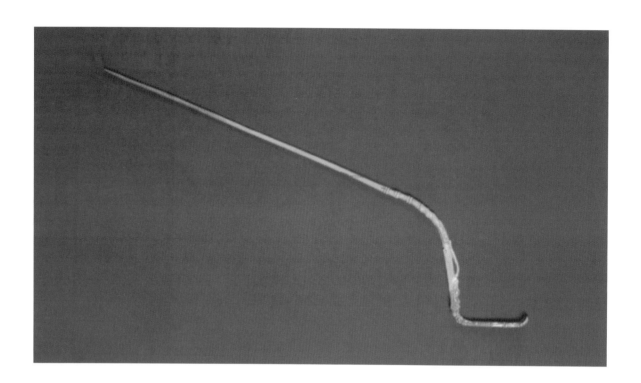

金耳扒

东晋

金质

长 23 厘米

Gold Ear Pick

Eastern Jin Dynasty

Gold

Length 23 cm

整体似一条腾云长龙，龙眼圆睁，龙嘴含珠。龙身刻画斜方格纹，龙尾呈卷曲状。顶端为扒勺。南京市栖霞区仙鹤观东晋高崧家族墓出土。

南京市博物馆藏

The gold ear pick looks like a long dragon with a coiled tail. The dragon has widely-opened eyes and a pearl in its mouth. Its body is covered with diamond patterns. The tip of the pick was used for picking ears. The artifact was unearthed from Gao Song's family tomb in Crane Daoist Temple in Xixia District, Nanjing City.

Preserved in Nanjing Municipal Museum

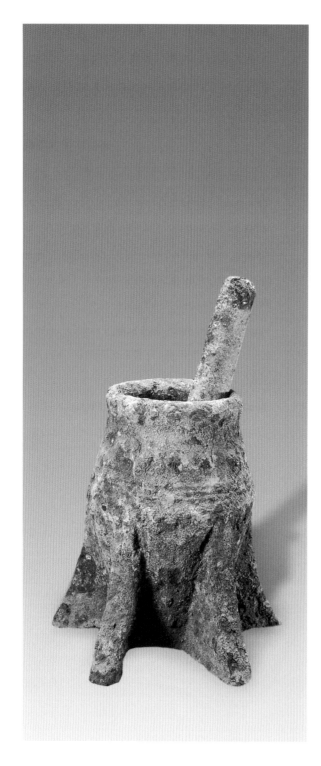

药臼（附杵）

晋

铁质

臼：口径 10 厘米，腹围 45 厘米，高 23.5 厘米

杵：长 30 厘米，直径 3 厘米

Iron Medicine Mortar and Pestle

Jin Dynasty

Iron

Mortar: Mouth Diameter 10 cm/ Belly Diameter

45 cm/ Height 23.5 cm

Pestle: Length 30 cm/ Diameter 3 cm

臼鼓腹，蹼足，腹有三道环纹。杵呈棒状。捣碎药物用。1989 年陕西省澄城县善化乡采集。

陕西医史博物馆藏

The mortar has a bugled belly with three raised rings and stands on web-shaped feet. The pestle is rod-shaped. The mortar and pestle was utilized for pounding drugs. It was collected in Shanhua Village of Chengcheng County, Shaanxi Province, in 1989.

Preserved in Shaanxi Museum of Medical History

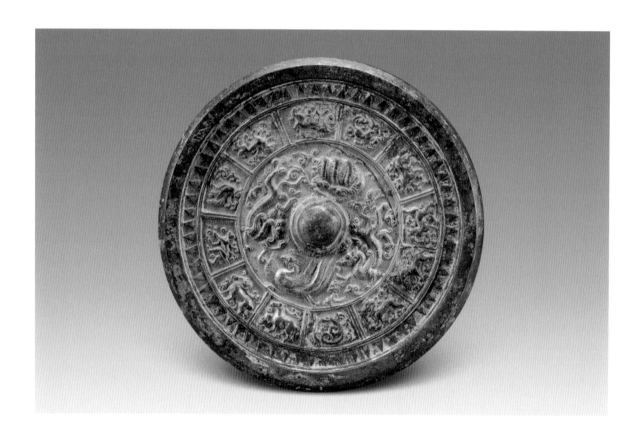

十二生肖四神镜

北朝

铜质

直径 16.9 厘米

Mirror of Chinese Zodiacs and the Four Gods

Northern Dynasty

Bronze

Diameter 16.9 cm

圆形。圆钮，圆钮座。钮座外环布浮雕青龙、白虎、朱雀、玄武四神；在双线界格内环雕十二生肖像，其外饰锯齿纹一周。河南省洛阳市庞家沟出土。

洛阳博物馆藏

The mirror itself, its knob and the knob base are all circular. The Four Gods (Green Dragon, White Tiger, Red Phoenix, and Black Tortoise) in relief surround the knob base. Outside the Four Gods are the twelve Chinese zodiacs surrounded by a ring of dented patterns. The mirror was unearthed in Pangjiagou of Luoyang City, Henan Province.

Preserved in Luoyang Museum

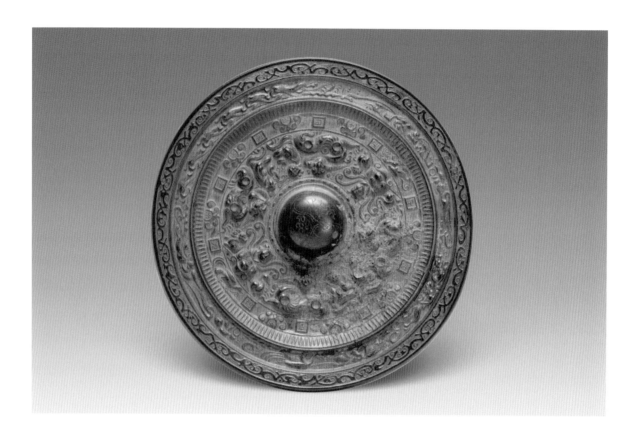

鎏金九子神兽镜

南朝

铜质

直径 13.6 厘米

Gilt Mirror of Supernatural Animals

Southern Dynasty

Bronze

Diameter 13.6 cm

圆形。圆钮，钮面有错金兽纹，连珠纹钮座。
镜背鎏金，内区纹饰为东王公、西王母及神
兽，其外有方枚与半圆相间环列，方枚上有
铭文。外区饰神人、龙、凤及神兽，边缘饰
云纹一周。1971年湖北省鄂城544工地出土。

湖北省博物馆藏

This circular mirror has a hemispherical knob
with animal patterns in gold inlay on it. The
knob base is decorated with a ring of pearl
patterns. The reverse side of the mirror is gilt.
The principal motifs consist of two segments.
In the inner segment there are the King of the
East, the Queen of the West, and supernatural
animals surrounded by squares and semicircles
arranged alternately. Inscriptions are in the
squares. Patterns in the outer segment include
supernatural beings, dragons, phoenixes,
and other supernatural animals. The edge is
decorated with cloud patterns. The mirror
was unearthed at No. 544 Construction Site in
Echeng, Hubei Province, in 1971.
Preserved in Hubei Museum

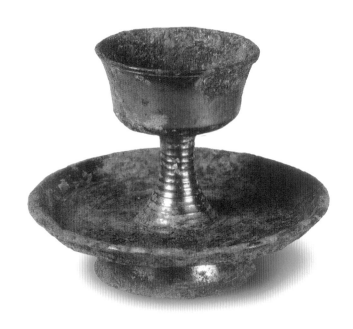

铜灯

南朝

铜质

口径 7.4 厘米，底径 6.5 厘米，通高 10.3 厘米

灯盏：高 4.3 厘米，壁厚 0.2~0.3 厘米，插柄长 2.8 厘米

插座：盘径 14 厘米，灯盘高 1.2 厘米，上径 2.1 厘米，下径 4.3 厘米，高 3.8 厘米，圈足高 2 厘米

Copper Lamp

Southern Dynasty

Bronze

Mouth Diameter 7.4 cm/ Bottom Diameter 6.5 cm/ Total Height 10.3 cm

Lamp: Height 4.3 cm/ Thickness 0.2–0.3 cm/ Stem Length 2.8 cm

Plate: Diameter 14 cm/ Height 1.2 cm/ Upper Diameter 2.1 cm/ Lower Diameter 4.3 cm/ Height 3.8 cm/ Base Height 2 cm

铜灯由灯盏和灯座组成。灯盏杯形，侈口，束腰，下有插柄。灯座含插座、灯盘和圈足。插座倒喇叭形，饰 13 道竹节纹；灯盘侈口，小唇边弧腹；圈足外撇。通体素面，盏杯口内外各饰一道弦纹，灯盘内饰三道弦纹。器表未锈蚀部分黑而发亮。1993 年江苏省江都市（今扬州市江都区）出土。

扬州市江都博物馆藏

The lamp consists of an upper lamp and a lower part. The upper lamp is in the shape of a cup with a wide flared mouth and a contracted belly. On each side of its rim, there is a ring of raised line. The lower part is composed of a stem, a plate, and a base. The stem, which resembles an inverted trumpet, is decorated with thirteen bamboo-joint patterns. The concave plate has three raised rings on its surface. The part of the lamp not covered with rust is still shiny. The lamp was unearthed in Jiangdu City (Now Jiangdu District of Yangzhou City), Jiangsu Province, in 1993.

Preserved in Jiangdu Museum of Yangzhou City

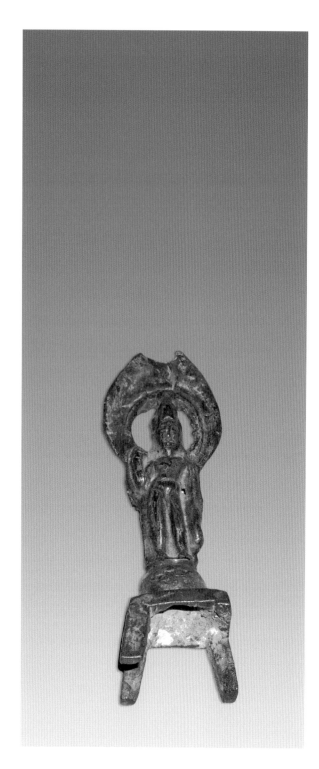

铜佛像

六朝

铜质

宽 2.2 厘米，高 8 厘米，重 50 克

Copper Buddha Figurine

Six Dynasties

Bronze

Width 2.2 cm/ Height 8 cm/ Weight 50 g

方底座，立佛，头上饰一圈佛光。有残。陕西
省咸阳市秦都区征集。

陕西医史博物馆藏

The Buddha figurine stands on a square base.
Surrounding the Buddha's head is a circle of
flammule, which is incomplete. The artifact
was collected in Qindu District, Xianyang City,
Shaanxi Province.

Preserved in Shaanxi Museum of Medical History

◈ 第二章　隋唐五代

Chapter Two　Sui, Tang, and Five Dynasties

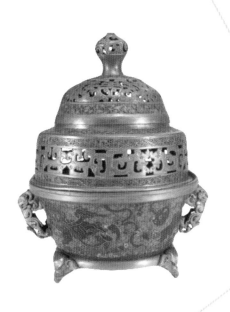

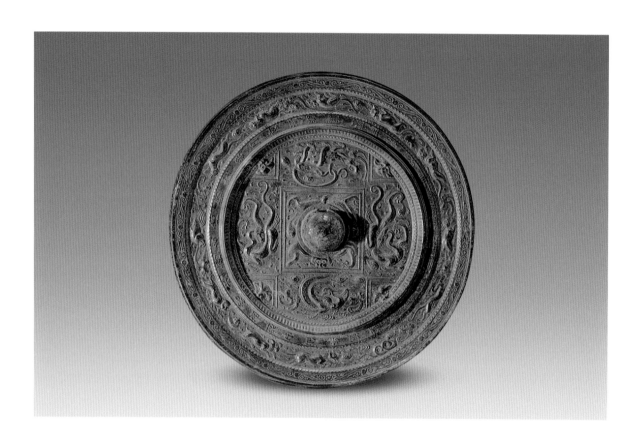

仙山并照四神镜

隋

铜质

直径 22 厘米

Mirror of the Four Supernatural Beasts

Sui Dynasty

Bronze

Diameter 22 cm

圆形。圆钮，伏兽纹钮座。钮座外双线方格，方格四角与 "V" 形纹相对，划分四个纹饰区， "V" 形纹内各置一兽面。纹饰区内分别配置四灵。中区有铭文 "仙山并照，智水齐名……" 三十二字。外区环绕十二生肖。镜缘为几何形云纹。1955 年湖南省长沙市出土。

湖南省博物馆藏

This circular mirror has a hemispherical knob with a knob base decorated with crouching beasts. Outside the base is a square, across each corner of which there is a V-shaped design. There is an animal's face in each V-shaped design. The main motifs are separated into four segments. The inner segment is the Four Supernatural Beasts. The middle segment consists of 32 inscriptions about the theme of the mirror. There are the Chinese zodiacs in the outermost segment. The edge of the mirror is patterned with geometric cloud designs. The mirror was unearthed in Changsha, Hunan Province, in 1955.

Preserved in Hunan Provincial Museum

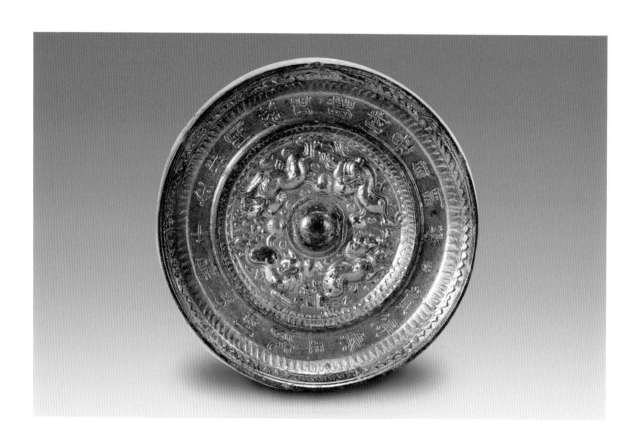

赏得秦王神兽镜

隋

铜质

直径 12 厘米

Mirror of Supernatural Beasts

Sui Dynasty

Bronze

Diameter 12 cm

圆形。圆钮，圆钮座。主题纹饰为四神兽，间以云纹。外圈为铭文一周二十字"赏得秦王镜，判不惜千金。非开欲照瞻，特是自明心"。1988 年陕西省长安县（今长安区）南里王村出土。

陕西省考古研究院藏

The circular mirror has a hemispherical knob sitting on a circular base. Its major motifs are the four supernatural beasts interspersed with cloud patterns. Around the main motifs are 20 inscriptions about the function of the mirror. The mirror was unearthed at Nanliwang Village, Chang'an District (now Chang'an District)of Xi'an City, Shaanxi Province, in 1988.

Preserved in Shaanxi Provincial Institute of Archaeology

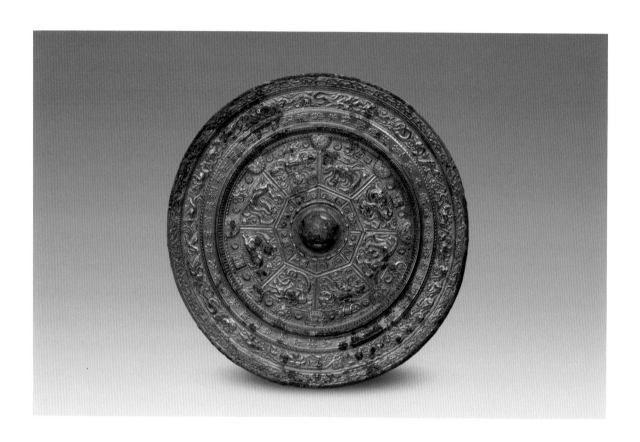

淮南起照神兽镜

隋

铜质

直径 25 厘米

Mirror of Supernatural Animals

Sui Dynasty

Bronze

Diameter 25 cm

圆形。圆钮，八角形钮座。其边棱皆双线，
八个凸起的方块上各镌一字。内区饰东王公、
西王母、四神及神兽，以双线相隔。外区饰
铭文一周及十二生肖等图案。边缘饰缠枝纹
一周。此镜纹饰繁复，制作精良。1978 年陕
西省永寿县出土。

陕西历史博物馆藏

The circular mirror has a hemispherical knob
sitting on an octagonal base. Its major motifs
consist of eight figures including the King
of the East, the Queen of the West, the Four
Supernatural Beasts, and other nameless
supernatural animals. Inscriptions and the
Chinese zodiacs surround the main motifs. This
delicate mirror with complicated decorative
patterns was unearthed in Yongshou County,
Shaanxi Province, in 1978.

Preserved in Shaanxi History Museum

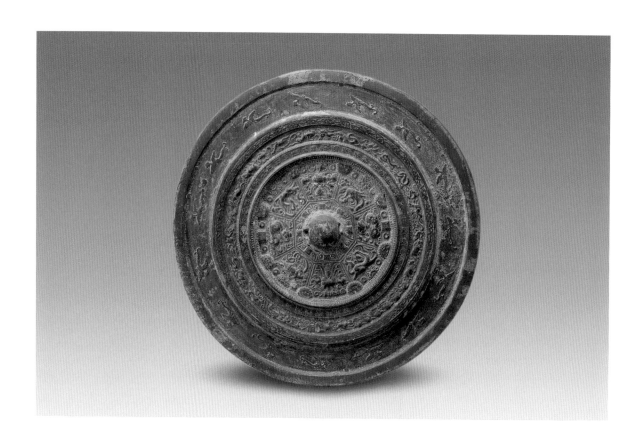

淮南起照八兽镜

隋

铜质

直径 33 厘米

Mirror of Eight Animals

Sui Dynasty

Bronze

Diameter 33 cm

圆形。圆钮，其边勾画八角形双线，线内铸有涡纹和方形字印。内区饰四神和东王公、西王母，外围有"宜君大吉"印记和圆圈纹。外区依次排列绳纹、铭文、十二生肖、水藻、鸾凤等各一圈。据铭文可证此镜系隋仁寿年间（601—604）在淮南一带制作而成。河南省洛阳市出土。

洛阳博物馆藏

The mirror is circular. Its hemispherical knob sets on an octagonal base with decorations of squares and scroll patterns. The principal motifs can be divided into two segments. Its inner segment consists of the Four Supernatural Beasts, the King of the East, and the Queen of the West, which are embraced by inscriptions of four words "Yi Jun Da Ji" (meaning wishing you extremely lucky) and ring patterns. The outer segment is composed of rings of string patterns, inscriptions, the Chinese zodiacs, waterweeds, and phoenixes. According to its inscriptions, this mirror was made in the region south of Huai River during Renshou Period (601–604) of the Sui Dynasty. It was unearthed in Luoyang City, Henan Province.
Preserved in Luoyang Museum

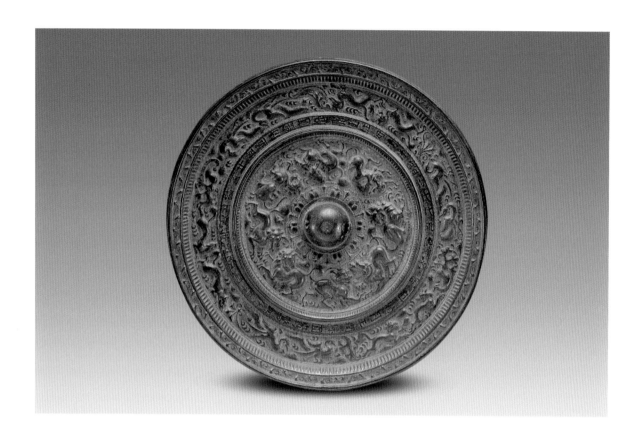

明逾满月神兽镜

隋

铜质

直径 24.3 厘米

Mirror of Supernatural Animals

Sui Dynasty

Bronze

Diameter 24.3 cm

圆形。圆钮，莲瓣纹钮座。内区环饰八狻猊，外圈有铭文一周；外区饰神兽呈奔跑追逐状。镜缘饰卷云纹。

四川博物院藏

The mirror is round with a hemispherical knob whose base is lotus-shaped. Its main motifs are separated by a ring of inscriptions. There are eight lions in the inner segment while the outer segment is decorated with running supernatural animals. The edge of the mirror is patterned with cirrus cloud designs.

Preserved in Sichuan Museum

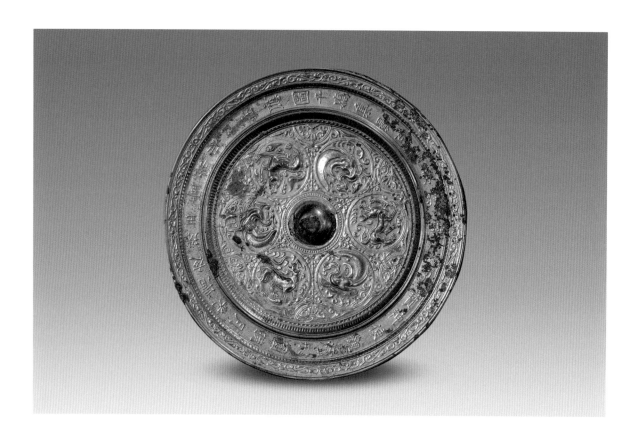

灵山孕宝神兽镜

隋

铜质

直径 17 厘米

Mirror of Supernatural Animals

Sui Dynasty

Bronze

Diameter 17 cm

圆形。圆钮，连珠纹钮座。内区有六团花，内置
三鸾鸟和三独角兽。外区镌铭文"灵山孕宝，神
使观炉……"一周六十四字。镜缘饰忍冬纹。

上海博物馆藏

The round mirror has a hemispherical knob with
a base decorated with a ring of pearl pattern.
The back of the mirror is composed of two main
segments. The inner segment consists of six
clusters of flowers, each one having a phoenix or
a unicorn inside. In its outer segment there is a
circle of 64 inscriptions. The edge is decorated with
honeysuckle designs.

Preserved in Shanghai Museum

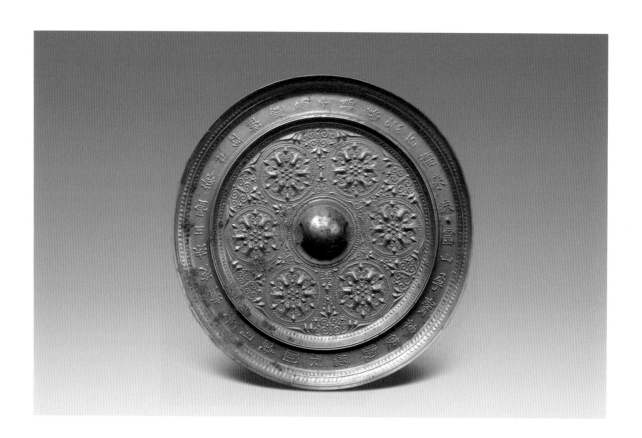

灵山孕宝团花镜

隋

铜质

直径 18.1 厘米

Mirror of Clustered Flowers

Sui Dynasty

Bronze

Diameter 18.1 cm

圆形。圆钮，连珠纹钮座。内区饰六朵团花，其间饰忍冬纹。外区内侧饰"灵山孕宝，神使观炉，形圆晓月，光清夜珠……"铭文一周。边缘饰锯齿纹。1981 年陕西省西安市出土。

陕西历史博物馆藏

The round mirror has a hemispherical knob whose base is decorated with a ring of pearl patterns. The inner segment is decorated with six flowers interspersed with honeysuckle designs. Inside the outer segment is a circle of inscriptions about the theme of the mirror. Its rim is decorated with dented patterns. The mirror was unearthed in Xi'an, Shaanxi Province, in 1981.

Preserved in Shaanxi History Museum

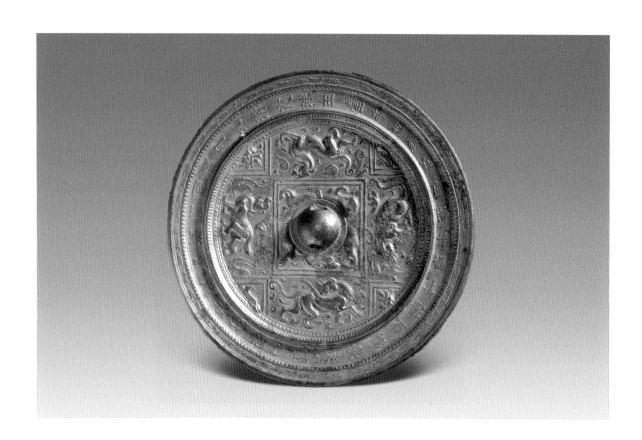

灵山孕宝四灵镜

隋

铜质

直径 18.5 厘米

Mirror of Four Supernatural Beasts

Sui Dynasty

Bronze

Diameter 18.5 cm

圆形。圆钮，卷草纹钮座。外有双线方栏，小连珠纹和栉纹带两周将镜背纹饰分成内外两区。内区方栏四角与"V"形纹对应，把内区又分割成四区，每区内各饰一神兽，有的昂首，有的回顾，均呈翘尾奔跑状。外区有铭文一周三十二字，铭文外有连珠纹和卷草纹各一周。

中国国家博物馆藏

This round mirror has a hemispherical knob sitting on a square base decorated with scroll designs. Outside the knob is a square, across each corner of which there is a V-shaped design. Its principal motifs are divided into two segments separated by a ring of pearl designs and a circle of comb designs. In the inner segment there are supernatural beasts with different postures. The outer segment has a circle of 32 inscriptions surrounded by a ring of pearl patterns and a circle of scroll designs.
Preserved in National Museum of China

铜镜

隋

铜质

直径 13.2 厘米，厚 0.5 厘米，重 300 克

圆形。圆钮。内区为海马图案，外区为三道圆环，边沿凸起。为生活用器，略有残损。陕西历史博物馆调拨。

陕西医史博物馆藏

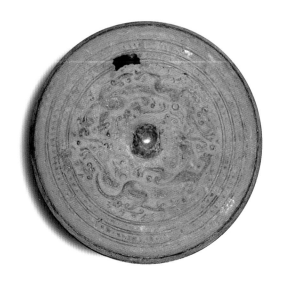

Bronze Mirror

Sui Dynasty

Bronze

Diameter 13.2 cm/ Thickness 0.5 cm/ Weight 300 g

The round mirror has a hemispherical knob. In its inner region there are the motifs of sea horses while in the outer region there are three raised rings. The mirror, a utensil for daily use, is slightly damaged. It was allocated from Shaanxi History Museum.

Preserved in Shaanxi Museum of Medical History

铜镜

唐

铜质

直径 4.8 厘米，厚 0.1 厘米，重 50 克

圆形。桥形钮。钮外一周分布浮雕瑞兽图案，已
模糊不清。边沿扁平。为生活用器。陕西省西安
市鄠邑区征集。

陕西医史博物馆藏

Bronze Mirror

Tang Dynasty

Bronze

Diameter 4.8 cm/ Thickness 0.1 cm/ Weight 50 g

The round mirror has a knob in the shape of a
bridge. Around the knob are indistinct auspicious
animals in relief. This mirror, which was a utensil
for daily use, was collected in Huyi District Shaanxi
Province.

Preserved in Shaanxi Museum of Medical History

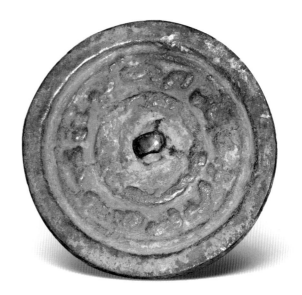

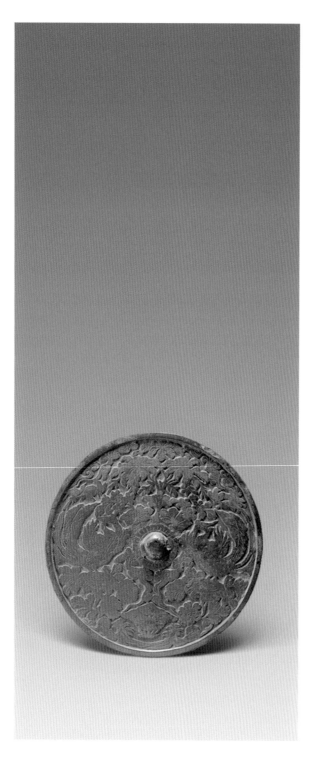

双凤牡丹镜

唐

铜质

直径 17.8 厘米

圆形。圆钮，花瓣钮座。钮外围剔地平雕双凤与牡丹花，纹饰左右对称。双凤相对站立于牡丹花上，呈展翅翘尾状。其间饰以阔叶折枝花、云纹及飞鸟纹。

陕西历史博物馆藏

Mirror Patterned with Phoenixes and Peonies

Tang Dynasty

Bronze

Diameter 17.8 cm

The round mirror has a hemispherical knob which sits on a flower-shaped knob base. Phoenixes and peonies are the principal motifs. The two phoenixes are resting on peonies, expending their wings and tails. The main motifs are interspersed with designs of plucked branches, clouds, and flying birds.

Preserved in Shaanxi History Museum

铜镜

唐

铜质

边长 10 厘米，重 150 克

"亞"字形。圆钮。钮外围浮雕花卉图案。为生活器具。内蒙古自治区达拉特旗征集。

陕西医史博物馆藏

Bronze Mirror

Tang Dynasty

Bronze

Side Length 10 cm/ Weight 150 g

The mirror is in the shape of the Chinese character "亞". Its hemispherical knob is surrounded by patterns of flowers in relief. The mirror, which was a utensil for daily use, was collected in Inner Mongolia Autonomous Region.

Preserved in Shaanxi Museum of Medical History

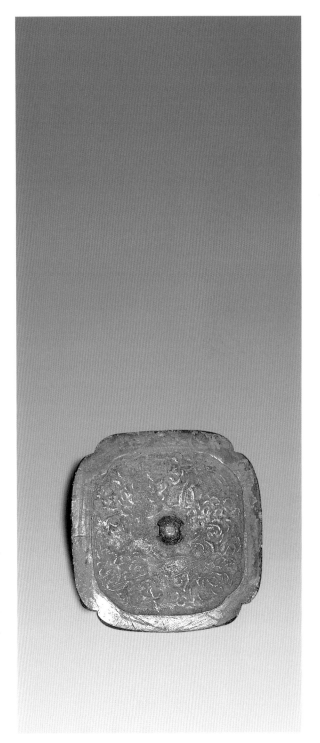

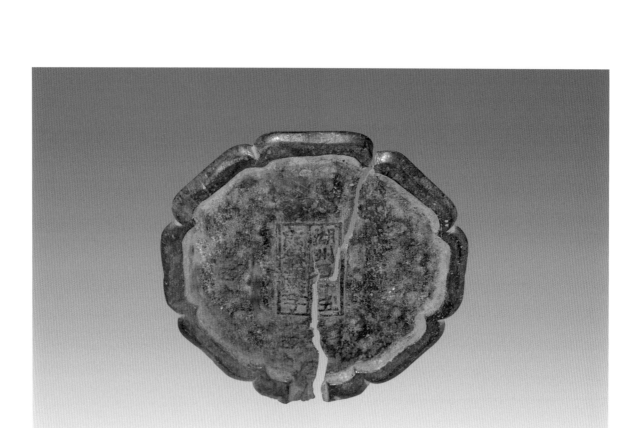

铜镜

唐

铜质

直径 11.7 厘米，重 150 克

Bronze Mirror

Tang Dynasty

Bronze

Diameter 11.7 cm/ Weight 150 g

八瓣葵花形，呈扁圆状，无纹饰，中部有铭文。

为生活器具，碎裂成两半。

陕西医史博物馆藏

The oblate mirror is in the shape of a mallow flower with eight petals and inscriptions in the center. It was a utensil for daily use and was broken into two pieces.

Preserved in Shaanxi Museum of Medical History

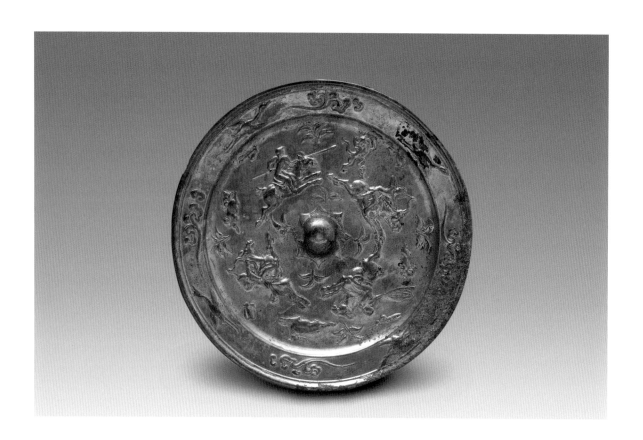

狩猎纹镜

唐

铜质

直径 14.9 厘米

Bronze Mirror Patterned with Hunting Scenes

Tang Dynasty

Bronze

Diameter 14.9 cm

圆形。圆钮，菱花钮座。饰四组狩猎纹。猎手纵马持长矛、弓箭、套索，马前为奔逃的野猪、鹿、兔和怪兽。主纹间饰蜂、蝶、折枝花，外缘饰一周云鹤纹。1955 年陕西省西安市出土。

陕西历史博物馆藏

The circular mirror has a hemispherical knob. Four sets of hunting scenes are decorated at its back. Hunters on horseback holding a spear, a bow or a lasso are chasing a wild pig, a deer, a rabbit and another beast which are running. Other designs include bees and butterflies, and plucked branches. Around the edge of the mirror there are crane designs. The mirror was unearthed in Xi'an, Shaanxi Province, in 1955.

Preserved in Shaanxi History Museum

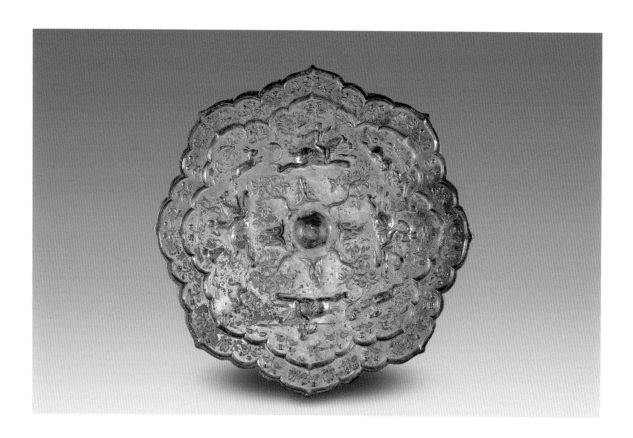

狩猎纹菱花镜

唐

铜质

直径 29 厘米

Linghua-shaped Mirror Patterned with Hunting Scene

Tang Dynasty

Bronze

Diameter 29 cm

八瓣菱花形。圆钮。以钮为中心置四株树木
和四座山峦。山树周围饰四组策马奔驰的狩
猎纹，或持长矛，或搭弓射箭，或回首观望，
马前有飞跑的兔、野猪、鹿和怪兽，并间以蜂、
蝶、雀鸟、蜻蜓、折枝花。镜缘饰折枝花和
蜂蝶一周。此镜表现手法写实，场面生动。
1961 年河南省洛阳市扶沟出土。

河南博物院藏

The mirror was made in the shape of
linghua flower with eight petals. Four trees
and mountains are arranged around the
hemispherical knob. Outside them are four
hunters with a spear or a bow riding on a horse.
The hunters are interspersed with a rabbit, a
boar, a deer, and a nameless animal. Patterns of
birds, bees, butterflies, dragonflies, and plucked
branches were also used to decorate the mirror.
The hunting scene was depicted realistically
and vividly. The mirror was unearthed in Fugou
of Luoyang City, Henan Province, in 1961.
Preserved in Henan Museum

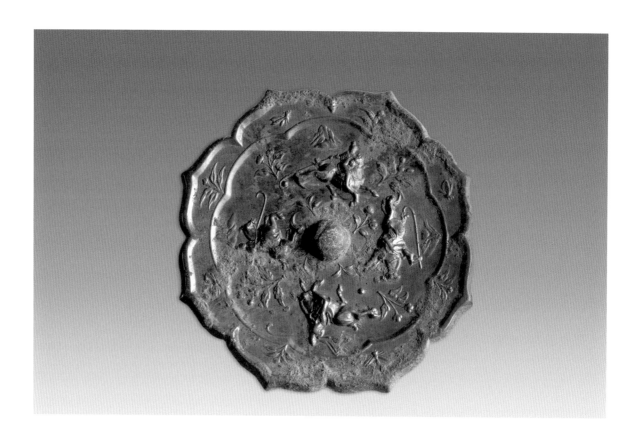

打马球菱花镜

唐

铜质

直径 11.3 厘米

Linghua-shaped Mirror with Polo-playing Scene

Tang Dynasty

Bronze

Diameter 11.3 cm

八瓣菱花形。圆钮。内区以钮为中心，饰四人骑马打球纹，或策马回首击球，或举踘杖追球，或俯身向前，场面紧张激烈。马侧饰山峦和折枝花。镜缘饰蜂、蝶和折枝花。此镜反映了当时社会生活的一个侧面。

故宫博物院藏

The mirror is in the shape of linghua flower with eight petals. Its principal motif is a scene of four people playing polo with a hemispherical knob as the center. The players are either hitting the ball with a bat or chasing the ball, which makes a vivid picture. Hills and flowers decorate the side of the horses while butterflies and flowers decorate the rim. This scene reflects one aspect of the life during the Tang Dynasty.
Preserved in The Palace Museum

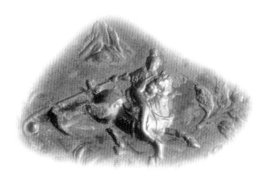

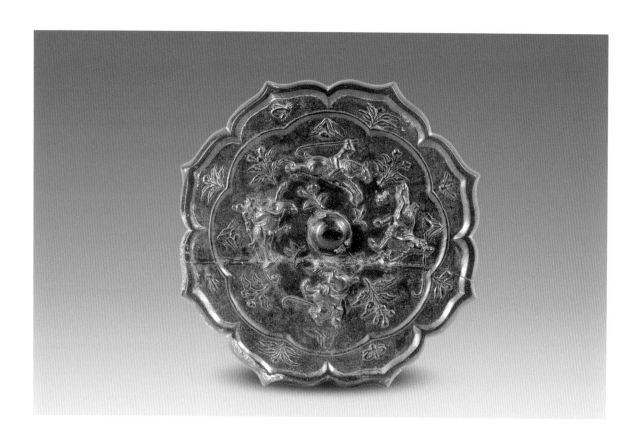

打马球菱花镜

唐

铜质

直径 19.4 厘米

Linghua-shaped Mirror with Polo-playing Scene

Tang Dynasty

Bronze

Diameter 19.4 cm

八瓣菱花形。圆钮。主纹为打马球图，四人骑马打击二球，一马四蹄腾空，骑者高举鞠仗由后前击；一马后蹄高扬，骑者横仗回击；一马前蹄腾空，骑者执仗前夺；一马昂首嘶鸣，骑者侧身执仗钩球。画面表现了马球比赛的激烈场面，与唐人的诗文记载相映成趣。1984 年安徽省怀宁县雷埠乡出土。

怀宁县文物管理所藏

The mirror is in the shape of linghua flower with eight petals. Its knob is hemispherical. The main motif is a scene of four people playing polo. The first horse is galloping with its hooves barely touching the ground while the rider is holding the bat high about to hit the ball. The second horse is rearing up. The third one is running with its forehooves hardly touching the ground and its rider is scrambling for the ball. The fourth horse is neighing with a perked head and its rider hitting the ball. This scene shows a very tense polo game, which forms a delightful contrast with what poets in the Tang Dynasty depicted. The mirror was unearthed in Leipu County, Huaining City, Anhui Province, in 1984.
Preserved in Huaining County Administration Office of Cultural Relics

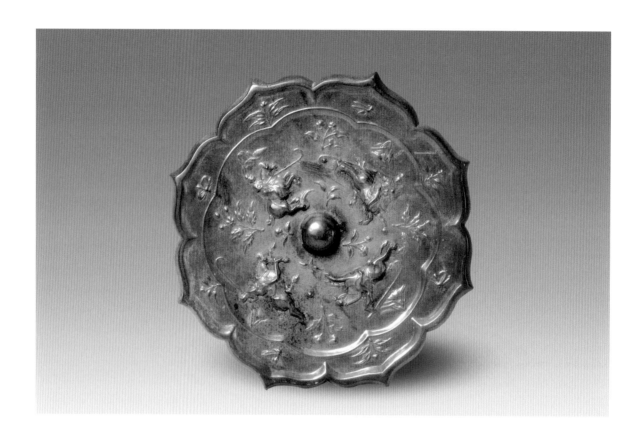

打马球铜镜

唐

铜质

直径 18.5 厘米，钮径 1 厘米

Bronze Mirror with Polo-playing Scene

Tang Dynasty

Bronze

Diameter 18.5 cm/ Knob Diameter 1 cm

八瓣菱花形。圆钮。镜背纹饰是四名骑士，手执鞠杖，跃马奔驰呈击球状；人与球之间衬以高山、花卉纹，显现出在郊外运动场比赛的情景。马球运动源于波斯，汉代传入我国，到了唐代，此运动十分活跃，深得皇帝和贵族的喜爱，成为铜镜纹饰的一种题材。目前我国仅存三面有关打马球图案的铜镜，以扬州出土的这面铜镜保存最好，是唐镜中的珍品。1965年邗江县（今江苏省扬州市邗江区）泰安乡金湾坝工地出土。

扬州博物馆藏

The mirror is in the shape of linghua flower with eight petals. Its knob is hemispherical. The main motif is a scene of four people on horseback playing polo. The players and the ball are separated by mountains and flower patterns, which presents the scene of playing the game on the outskirts. Only three mirrors with polo-playing scene have been preserved in China, and this mirror is the best conserved one. The mirror is a treasure among Tang Dynasty mirrors. It was unearthed at Jinwanba construction site in Hanjiang County(now Hanjiang District), Yangzhou City, Jiangsu Province, in 1965.

Preserved in Yangzhou Museum

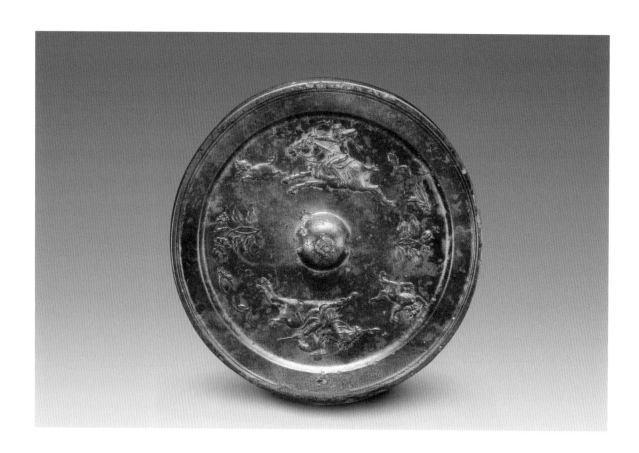

射猎纹铜镜

唐

铜质

直径 14.8 厘米

Bronze Mirror Patterned with Hunting Scene

Tang Dynasty

Bronze

Diameter 14.8 cm

圆形。圆钮。镜背采用浮雕，饰有两猎手骑在马背上
奔驰，手执弓箭、长枪，追逐着惊慌奔跑的野兽，其
间饰飞蝶和花木纹图案。画面中骑射者的描绘极具
动态感。

法国吉美国立亚洲艺术博物馆藏

The circular mirror has a hemispherical knob. At its back,
there are two hunters riding a galloping horse with bows
and spears in their hands while chasing the panicking
animals. Beside the hunters are butterflies and flower
patterns. All the designs are in relief. This artifact shows
a very vivid scene.

Preserved in Musée National des Arts Asiatiques-Guimet,
France

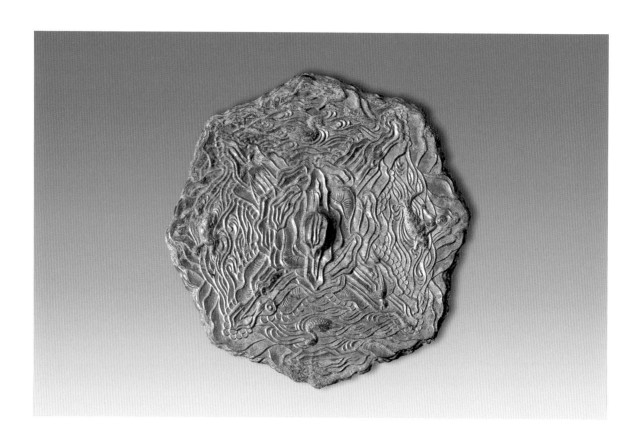

山海神人八角镜

唐

铜质

直径 17.7 厘米

Octagonal Mirror of Mountains, Seas and Immortals

Tang Dynasty

Bronze

Diameter 17.7 cm

八瓣菱花形。云纹钮，钮座为俯视的山岭，上有草。四角耸出四座各具形态的山峦，其中两山各有一飞禽展翅翱翔。山峦之间为波涛起伏的海水，有神禽异兽浮游其上，有一童子骑于鳌鱼上，这种鱼称龙鱼。整个图案云雾缭绕，山峦叠嶂，当取材于《山海经》故事。

日本千石唯司藏

The mirror is shaped like an eight-petaled flower. Its knob is decorated with cloud patterns and the knob base is decorated with mountains. Extending from each of the four corners is a mountain with a flying bird. Between mountains, there are choppy seas with water birds, fish and flying birds. A boy is sitting on supernatural fish which was named Dragon Fish. The motifs were based on stories in "Shan Hai Jing" (*Legends of Mountains and Seas*). Preserved in Sengoku Tadashi Museum, Japan

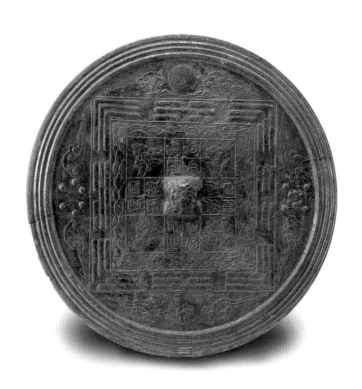

日月贞明八卦镜

唐

铜质

直径 25 厘米

Mirror of the Eight Diagrams

Tang Dynasty

Bronze

Diameter 25 cm

圆形。山形方钮。主题纹饰以八卦构成方框，四角饰山岳纹，相间四框内饰铭文："日月贞明，天地含为，写规万物，洞鉴百灵"。边缘饰日月星辰一周。此镜纹饰设计奇巧，寓容纳天地万物之意。河南省洛阳市磁涧出土。

洛阳博物馆藏

The mirror is circular and its square knob is made in the shape of a mountain. The pattern of the Eight Diagrams forms a square which embraces mountain patterns and inscriptions about the theme of the mirror. The whole square is surrounded by the sun, the moon, and stars. The elaborate design of the mirror implies embracing the universe. This mirror was unearthed in Cijian of Luoyang City, Henan Province.

Preserved in Luoyang Museum

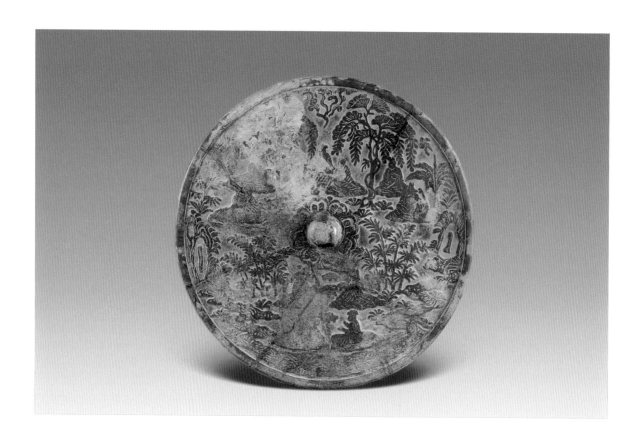

竹林七贤镜

唐

铜质

直径 21 厘米

Mirror of the Seven Sages of the Bamboo Grove

Tang Dynasty

Bronze

Diameter 21 cm

圆形。圆钮,莲花瓣钮座。主题纹饰为十一人,皆席地而坐。钮上方有两人对弈,一人静观,左侧两人坐于大树下,钮下方有四人交谈。其间饰山石、竹林、飞禽等。纹饰用浅浮雕手法,表现了竹林七贤的生活意境。1978年云南省大理市出土。

云南省博物馆藏

The mirror is round in shape. Its hemispherical knob has a lotus-shaped base. There are eleven people on the back of the mirror. On the top of the knob, two people are playing chess with another one watching. On the left of the knob, two people are sitting under a big tree while four people beneath the knob are chatting. All the major motifs in bas-relief are interspersed with mountains, bamboo groves, and flying birds. This mirror embodies the care-free life of the Seven Sages of the Bamboo Grove. It was unearthed in Dali, Yunnan Province, in 1978. Preserved in Yunnan Provincial Museum

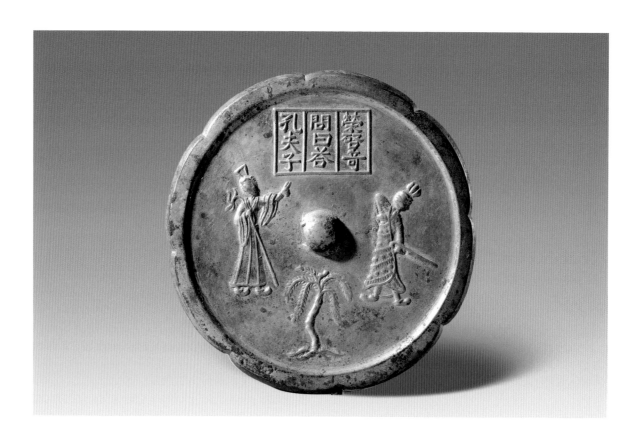

荣启奇葵花镜

唐

铜质

直径 12.9 厘米

Rong Qiqi Sunflower Mirror

Tang Dynasty

Bronze

Diameter 12.9 cm

八瓣葵花形。圆钮。钮左侧一人为孔子，顶冠着袍，左手前指，右手拄杖呈招呼状。右侧一人为荣启奇，高冠鹿裘，左手持琴，呈答言状。下面为一棵垂柳，上为"荣启奇问曰答孔夫子"的铭文。素凸缘。

洛阳博物馆藏

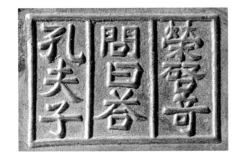

The mirror is in the shape of an eight-petaled mallow flower and its knob is hemispherical. The person on the left side of the knob is confucius pointing with his left hand and holding a stick in his right hand. The person on the right side is Rong Qiqi with his left hand holding a Qin, an ancient Chinese musical instrument. He is answering Confucius's question. Beneath the knob is a willow tree. Above the knob are nine inscriptions "Rong Qiqi Wen Yue Da Kong Fu Zi" (meaning Rong Qiqi is answering Confucius's question). The convex edge of the mirror is plain.

Preserved in Luoyang Museum

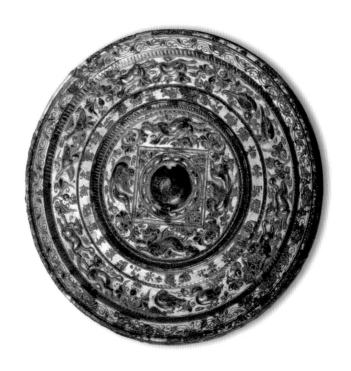

"鉴若止水" 镜

唐

铜质

直径 24.6 厘米，厚 1.7 厘米，重 4260 克

Mirror with Four Chinese Characters Reading "Jian Ruo Zhi Shui"

Tang Dynasty

Bronze

Diameter 24.6 cm/ Thickness 1.7 cm/ Weight 4,260 g

圆形。圆钮，方形钮座。钮座周围饰四兽纹，再向外围为一周铭文，再向外为一周浮雕禽兽纹，外缘为卷云纹。系章怀太子妃房氏生前所用之物。

乾陵博物馆藏

The mirror is round and has a hemispherical knob with a square base, which is surrounded by four supernatural animals. These animals are surrounded by a ring of inscriptions, then a ring of birds and animal patterns in relief, and a ring of cirrus cloud design even farther. The mirror belonged to the wife of Prince Zhanghuai during her life time.

Preserved in Qianling Museum

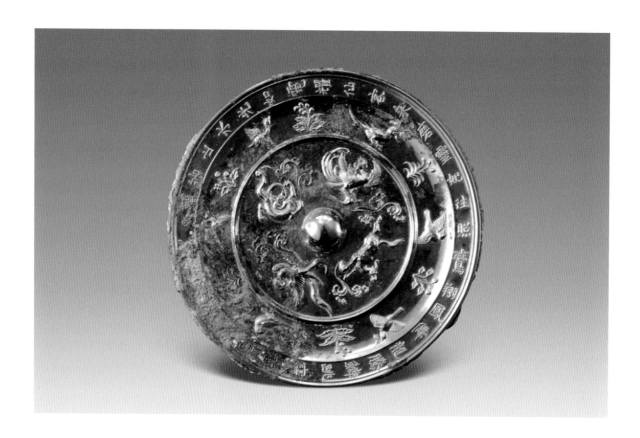

"鉴若止水"镜

唐

铜质

直径 20.4 厘米

Mirror with Four Chinese Characters Reading "Jian Ruo Zhi Shui"

Tang Dynasty

Bronze

Diameter 20.4 cm

圆形。圆钮，圆钮座。内区有两兽两鸟，呈蟠龙飞腾，麒麟跳跃飞奔，鸾鸟展翅飞翔，凤凰起舞状。外区六只鸾鸟，或憩息，或飞翔，其间饰花草纹。镜缘铭文一周三十二字。此镜内区所饰动物均一足镂空，颇为少见。

日本千石唯司藏

The mirror is round with a hemispherical knob sitting on a round base. There are four supernatural animals in the inner segment. They are a flying dragon, a leaping kylin, a flying bird, and a dancing phoenix. The outer segment consists of six birds flying or resting, interspersed with various flowers. There are thirty-two inscriptions on the edge of the back. One foot of each animal in the inner segment was hollowed out, which was very rare.

Preserved in Sengoku Tadashi Museum, Japan

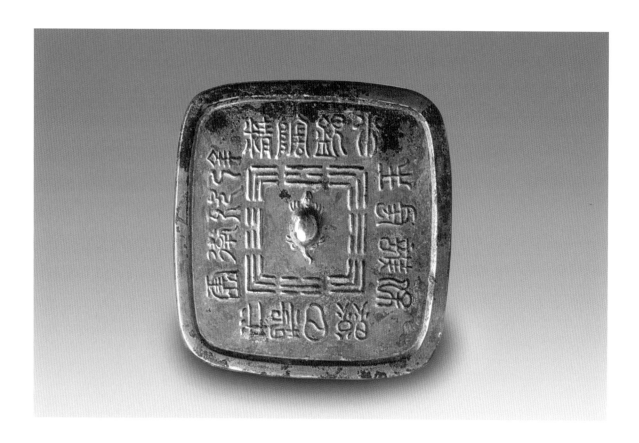

八卦铭文方镜

唐

铜质

边长 15.6 厘米

Square Mirror with Inscriptions and the Eight Diagrams

Tang Dynasty

Bronze

Side Length 15.6 cm

四方委角形。龟形钮。钮外方折环列八卦象，其外四边各有四字篆铭为："水银阴精，辟邪卫灵，形神日照，保护长生"素凸缘。

山西博物院藏

The mirror is in the shape of a square with rounded edges. Its knob, which resembles a turtle, is surrounded by the pattern of the Eight Diagrams. Outside it there are sixteen seal-script words with four on each side, which indicate the function of the mirror. The convex rim is plain.

Preserved in Shanxi Museum

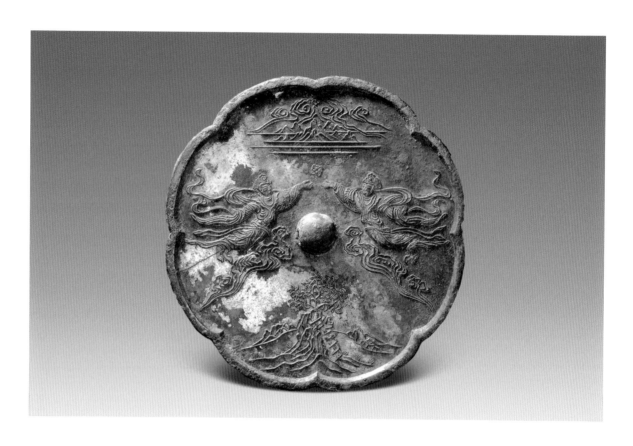

飞天葵花镜

唐

铜质

直径 25.3 厘米

Mallow Flower-shaped Mirror

Tang Dynasty

Bronze

Diameter 25.3 cm

八瓣葵花形。圆钮。钮两侧各一飞天，头戴宝冠，天衣飘逸，帔帛自然垂落，两飞天各举一手向上前方，共持一个四瓣花形物。飞天下方饰祥云，钮上方正中为四道横线，线上饰崇山峻岭，山头祥云环绕。钮下方饰山峰，峰顶生长枝叶繁茂的树木。1955年陕西省西安市出土。

中国国家博物馆藏

The mirror is in the shape of an eight-petaled mallow flower. The knob is hemispherical with an apsaras on its left side and right side, respectively. The two apsarases with a crown and their clothes floating in the wind are holding a flower together. Under their feet are auspicious clouds. In the center right above the knob are four horizontal lines, on which mountains are surrounded by clouds. Under the knob there is a mountain covered with luxuriant trees. The mirror was excavated in Xi'an, Shaanxi Province, in 1955.

Preserved in National Museum of China

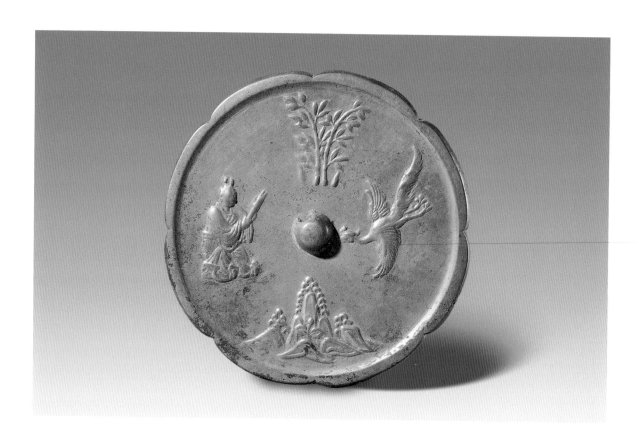

吹笙引凤葵花镜

唐

铜质

直径 12.9 厘米

Mallow Flower-shaped Mirror

Tang Dynasty

Bronze

Diameter 12.9 cm

八瓣葵花形。圆钮。钮左一人端坐吹笙，神情专注，右侧一凤展翅翘尾，闻声而至。上方为竹树一丛，下方为崇山峻岭。据《列仙传》载，吹笙者当为周灵王太子王子乔。此镜纹饰精练，生动地表现了吹笙引凤的主题。河南省洛阳市出土。

洛阳市文物工作队藏

The mirror is in the shape of an eight-petaled mallow flower and its knob is hemispherical. On the left side of the knob, a man is playing the Sheng, a reed pipe wind instrument, while on the right side a phoenix is flying towards him. A bamboo grove above and mountains below were also used to decorate the mirror. According to "Lie Xian Zhuan" (*Legends of the Immortals*), the person was Prince Qiao, the son of King Zhou Ling Wang. The scene vividly depicts the theme of playing the Sheng to attract the phoenix. The mirror was unearthed in Luoyang, Henan Province.

Collected by Luoyang Cultural Relics Work Team

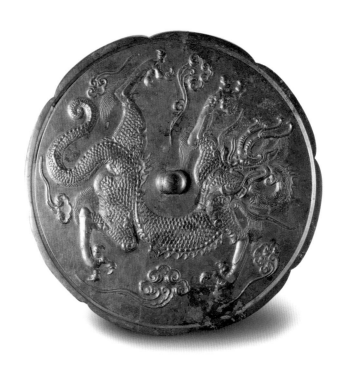

云龙纹葵花镜

唐

铜质

直径 24 厘米

Mallow Flower-shaped Mirror Patterned with Clouds and Dragon

Tang Dynasty

Bronze

Diameter 24 cm

八瓣葵花形。圆钮。镜背为一条盘龙，曲颈回顾，张口吐舌，周身饰鳞纹。龙体上下衬五朵流云，构图生动，制作精良。1984 年河南省偃师县（今偃师市）杏园出土。

中国社会科学院考古研究所藏

The mirror is in the shape of an eight-petaled mallow flower. Its knob is hemispherical. The principal motif is a dragon looking over its shoulders with its mouth wide open. The dragon's body is covered with scales. Five clouds surround the dragon. This well-made mirror was unearthed at Xingyuan site of Yanshi County (now Yanshi City), Henan Province, in 1984.

Preserved in the Institute of Archaeology, the Chinese Academy of Social Sciences

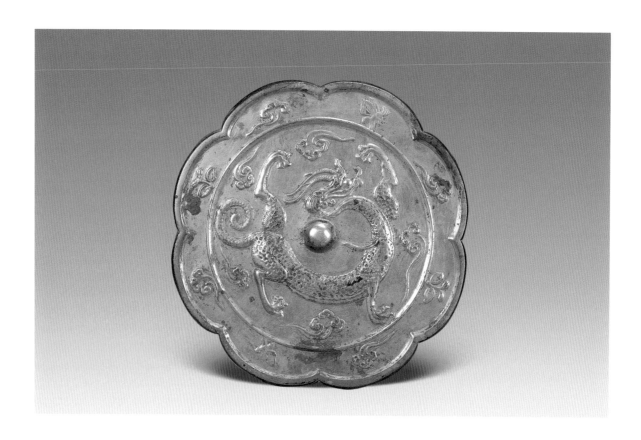

云龙纹葵花镜

唐

铜质

直径 20.5 厘米

Mallow Flower-shaped Mirror Patterned with Clouds and Dragon

Tang Dynasty

Bronze

Diameter 20.5 cm

八瓣葵花形。圆钮。龙首高仰，双角翘起，口衔宝珠，体躯盘曲，龙尾向上卷曲，两爪高高扬起，两爪屈伸。龙周围饰有流云。镜缘饰流云和折枝花。整个纹饰用浅浮雕表现，使龙更显气韵生动。河南省洛阳市北瑶出土。

洛阳博物馆藏

The mirror is in the shape of an eight-petaled mallow flower. Its knob is hemispherical. The principal motif is a dragon raising its head with its two claws holding high. The tortuous dragon has a pearl in its mouth. It is surrounded by cloud patterns. The edge of the mirror is decorated with designs of clouds and plucked branches. All the patterns are in bas-relief, which makes the dragon lively. The mirror was unearthed in Beiyao of Luoyang City, Henan Province.

Preserved in Luoyang Museum

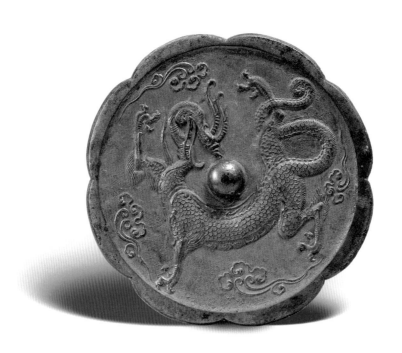

云龙纹葵花镜

唐

铜质

直径 12.9 厘米

Mallow Flower-shaped Mirror Patterned with Clouds and Dragon

Tang Dynasty

Bronze

Diameter 12.9 cm

八瓣葵花形。圆钮。主题纹饰为一龙呈昂首

飞腾状，龙身上的鳞纹清晰可辨，龙回首向

钮，呈口吞钮珠状。周围饰四朵祥云。

陕西历史博物馆藏

The mirror is made in the shape of an eight-petaled mallow flower. Its knob is hemispherical. The principal motif is a soaring dragon holding its head high. The dragon, with a pearl in its mouth, is looking back at the knob. The scales on its body are very clear. Four auspicious clouds surround the dragon.

Preserved in Shaanxi History Museum

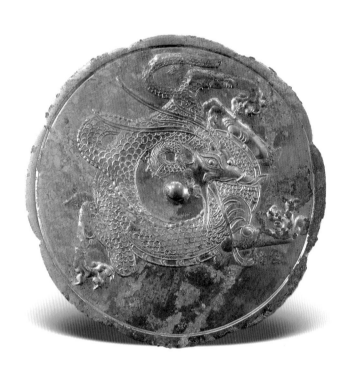

蟠龙纹葵花镜

唐

铜质

直径 27.4 厘米

Mallow Flower-shaped Mirror Patterned with Dragon

Tang Dynasty

Bronze

Diameter 27.4 cm

八瓣葵花形。圆钮。蟠龙为浅浮雕，龙头右向，双角分支呈飘举状，双目呈菱形，张口吐舌，舌甚长，龙体向右旋转呈圆形，四足雄健，爪勾曲有力，通体满饰鳞纹。此镜所饰龙纹形象特别，且镜体较大，是不可多得的珍品。

日本千石唯司藏

The mirror is in the shape of an eight-petaled mallow flower and has a hemispherical knob. Its back is decorated with a dragon in relief. The dragon has two long antlers, four forceful claws, and rhomb-shaped eyes. It opens its mouth wide, showing a long protruding tongue. Its body is covered with scales. The dragon rotates rightwards, forming a ball shape. The image of this dragon is quite lively and special and the mirror is quite big, which makes this artifact precious.

Preserved in Sengoku Tadashi Museum, Japan

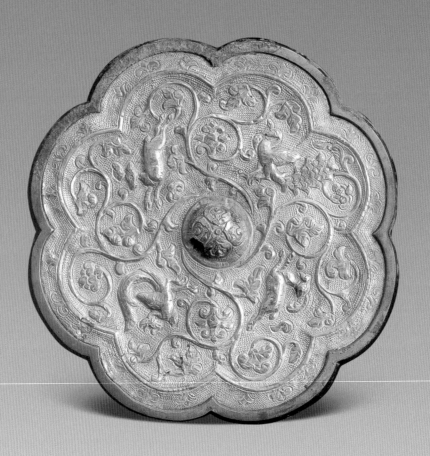

银背鎏金鸟兽葵花镜

唐

铜质

直径 14.6 厘米

八瓣葵花形。圆钮，圆钮座。钮周围环饰两鸟两兽。两鸟为凤凰，展翅争艳。两兽呈奔驰状，一兽为羊，双角翘起；一兽为鹿，角呈灵芝形。兽鸟间饰折枝花。外缘为花饰。纹饰以细珠纹为地，表面均鎏金。

日本千石唯司藏

Gilt Mallow Flower-shaped Mirror Patterned with Birds and Animals

Tang Dynasty

Bronze

Diameter 14.6 cm

The mirror is in the shape of an eight-petaled mallow flower. The hemispherical knob has a round base. The principal motifs are two birds and two animals. Two birds are phoenixes with outspread wings. The two running animals are a goat with perking horns and a deer with ganoderma-shaped antlers. The main patterns are interspersed with designs of plucked branches. The background is fine pearl designs. The mirror is gilt.

Preserved in Sengoku Tadashi Museum, Japan

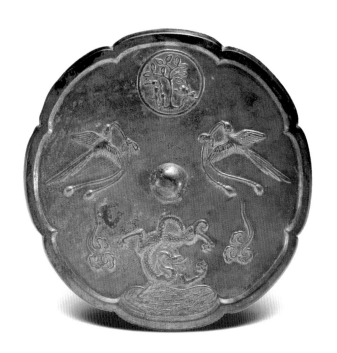

双鹊衔绶葵花镜

唐

铜质

直径 15.2 厘米

Mallow Flower-shaped Mirror of Double Magpies

Tang Dynasty

Bronze

Diameter 15.2 cm

八瓣葵花形。圆钮。镜钮两侧各饰一展翅飞翔的鹊鸟，口衔绶带。上方是月宫图，内有桂树、捣药的玉兔及蟾蜍。下方为蛟龙出海图，两边各有一朵祥云。四川省平武县城隍庙出土。

四川博物院藏

The mirror is in the shape of an eight-petaled mallow flower and has a hemispherical knob. The principal motifs are two flying magpies with a ribbon in their beaks. On the top of the two birds is a picture of the moon with a laurel tree, a toad, and a rabbit crushing herbal medicine. Under the magpies is a dragon jumping out of the sea. This mirror was unearthed in the City Temple of Pingwu County, Sichuan Province.
Preserved in Sichuan Museum

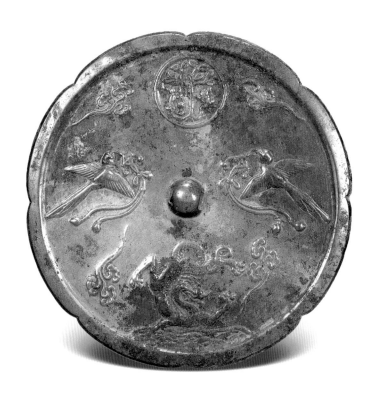

双鸾衔绶葵花镜

唐

铜质

直径 17.3 厘米

Mallow Flower-shaped Mirror of Double Magpies

Tang Dynasty

Bronze

Diameter 17.3 cm

八瓣葵花形。圆钮。主题纹饰为双鸾衔绶，凌空飞翔。上部饰月宫图，内有桂树、玉兔。下部饰巨龙腾跃出海，间饰祥云。河南省洛阳市洛阳矿山厂出土。

洛阳博物馆藏

The mirror is in the shape of an eight-petaled mallow flower and has a hemispherical knob. The principal motifs are two magpies flying in the sky with a ribbon in their beaks. On the top of the two birds is a picture of the moon with a laurel tree and a rabbit. Under the magpies is a dragon jumping out of the sea. Auspicious clouds intersperse the motifs. This mirror was unearthed at Kuangshanchang site of Luoyang City, Henan Province.

Preserved in Luoyang Museum

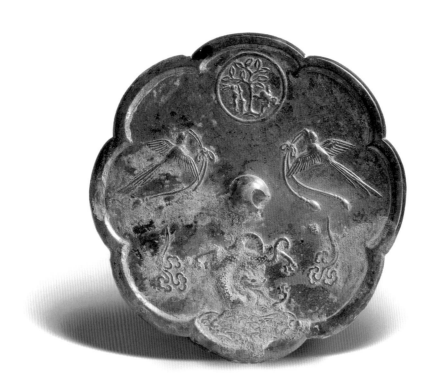

双鸾衔绶葵花镜

唐

铜质

直径 15.3 厘米

Mallow Flower-shaped Mirror of Double Mythical Birds

Tang Dynasty

Bronze

Diameter 15.3 cm

八瓣葵花形。桥形钮。纹饰可分为三组，上部为一满月，内有桂树、玉兔及蟾蜍。下部为一出水蛟龙，海面为波纹。两侧饰口衔绶带的鸾鸟，展翅凌空，相对飞翔。1983 年陕西省商县（今商洛市商州区）出土。

陕西历史博物馆藏

The mirror is in the shape of an eight-petaled mallow flower and has a hemispherical knob. The principal motifs are two mythical birds flying in the sky with a ribbon in their beaks. Above the two birds is the full moon with a laurel tree, a rabbit, and a toad. In the lower part of the mirror there is a dragon jumping out of the wavy sea. This mirror was unearthed in Shang County (now Shangzhou District of Shangluo City) Shaanxi Province, in 1983. Preserved in Shaanxi History Museum

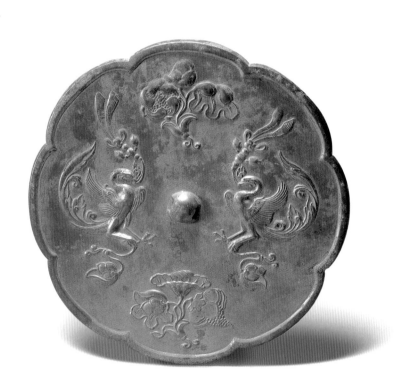

双鸾葵花镜

唐

铜质

直径 24 厘米

Mallow Flower-shaped Mirror of Double Mythical Birds

Tang Dynasty

Bronze

Diameter 24 cm

八瓣葵花形。圆钮。钮两侧各饰一鸾鸟相对
而立。鸾鸟口衔绶带，展翅欲翔，长尾上翘，
一爪踏于荷叶枝的莲蓬上。钮上、下各饰莲
花荷叶纹。陕西省西安市高楼村出土。

陕西历史博物馆藏

The mirror is in the shape of an eight-petaled
mallow flower and has a hemispherical knob.
The principal motifs are two mythical birds on
both sides of the knob. The birds, with tilting
tails, are resting on a lotus branch with a ribbon
in their beaks. There are patterns of lotus and
lotus leaves above and under the knob. The
mirror was unearthed at Gaolou Village of
Xi'an City, Shaanxi Province.

Preserved in Shaanxi History Museum

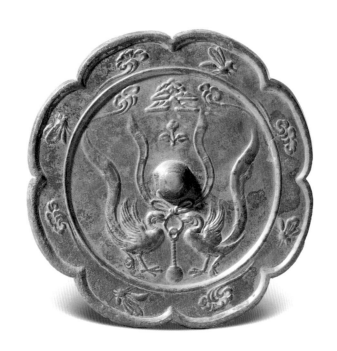

双鸾葵花镜

唐

铜质

直径 14.7 厘米

Mallow Flower-shaped Mirror of Double Mythical Birds

Tang Dynasty

Bronze

Diameter 14.7 cm

八瓣葵花形。圆钮。钮以上花枝云朵间饰山岳纹，钮以下饰双鸾相对衔绶，呈展翅翘尾状，绶带上飘。在凸弦纹与连弧镜边之间，饰蝴蝶及云纹相间环绕。河南省洛阳市关林3号墓出土。

洛阳博物馆藏

The mirror is in the shape of an eight-petaled mallow flower and has a hemispherical knob. Under the knob are two mythical birds facing each other with a ribbon in their beaks. There are patterns of clouds, a flower, and a mountain above the knob. The outer segment is decorated with butterflies and clouds. The mirror was unearthed from Tomb No. 3 at Guanlin site of Luoyang City, Henan Province.
Preserved in Luoyang Museum

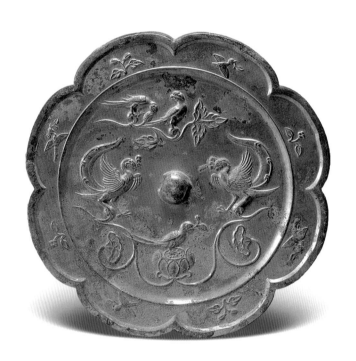

双鸾葵花镜

唐

铜质

直径 22 厘米

Mallow Flower-shaped Mirror of Double Mythical Birds

Tang Dynasty

Bronze

Diameter 22 cm

八瓣葵花形。圆钮。钮两侧各一鸾鸟立于花枝上，呈振翅翘尾状。钮上侧饰两鸟站于花枝上，一鸟啄葡萄，一鸟回首顾盼。钮下侧饰一鸟口衔花枝站于莲蓬上。边缘饰四只折枝花与四鸟相间环列。1956 年陕西省宝鸡市姜城堡出土。

陕西历史博物馆藏

The mirror is in the shape of an eight-petaled mallow flower and has a hemispherical knob. On the right side and the left side of the knob respectively a mythical bird is resting on a branch with its tail tilting upward. Another two birds are standing on a branch above the knob. One of them is pecking at grapes while the other is looking back. Beneath the knob, a bird is standing on a lotus seedpod with a flower in its beak. Four plucked branches and four birds alternately surround the main motifs along the edge of the mirror back. The mirror was unearthed at Jiangchengbao site of Baoji City, Shaanxi Province, in 1956.

Preserved in Shaanxi History Museum

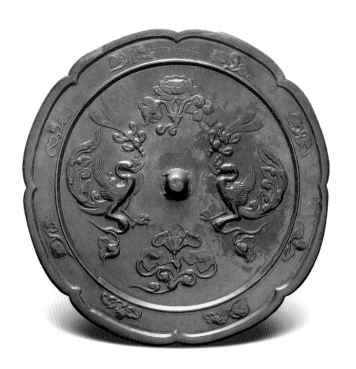

双鸾葵花镜

唐

铜质

直径 24.4 厘米

Mallow Flower-shaped Mirror of Double Birds

Tang Dynasty

Bronze

Diameter 24.4 cm

八瓣葵花形。圆钮，无钮座。纹饰由一道凸弦纹将镜背纹饰分成内外二区。内区饰双鸾鸟对称而立，鸾鸟屈颈挺胸，双翅伸展，长尾上翘，口衔绶带，一足凌空，一足踏于花枝上。上下方各饰花枝，均为两片花叶托起盛开的花朵，形态各异。外区饰单双叶花枝相间排列。镜体厚重，宽边缘。

中国国家博物馆藏

The mirror is in the shape of an eight-petaled mallow flower and has a hemispherical knob without a base. A raised ring divides the patterns into two segments. In the inner segment there are a pair of standing birds. They are expanding their wings and standing on a branch on one leg, with a ribbon in their beaks. There is a branch with a blooming flower above and under the knob respectively. The outer segment is decorated with branches and flowers arranged alternately.

Preserved in National Museum of China

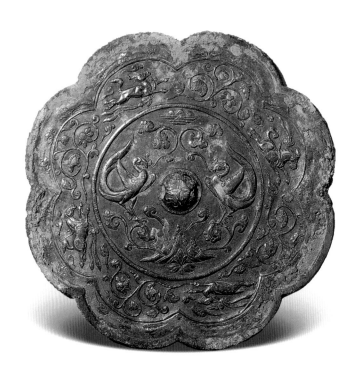

银背鎏金双鸟葵花镜

唐

铜质

直径 24.5 厘米

Gilt Mallow Flower-shaped Mirror of Double Phoenixes

Tang Dynasty

Bronze

Diameter 24.5 cm

八瓣葵花形。伏兽钮，连珠纹钮座。钮两侧为凤鸟，均展翅舒尾而舞，上下饰灵山与蔓枝，外区饰二天马、一鹿、一麒麟，呈奔驰飞翔状，间饰花草纹。纹饰表面均鎏金，但大多脱落。

日本泉屋博古馆藏

The mirror is in the shape of an eight-petaled mallow flower and has a knob shaped like a crouching animal. The knob base is decorated with pearl designs. On both sides of the knob there are two dancing phoenixes with expanded wings and tails. Mountains and branches are arranged between the two birds. The outer segment is patterned with two Pegasuses, one deer and one kylin, which are interspersed with patterns of flowers and grass. The surface used to be gilt, but most part of it has shedded.

Preserved in Sen-oku Hakuko Kan, Japan

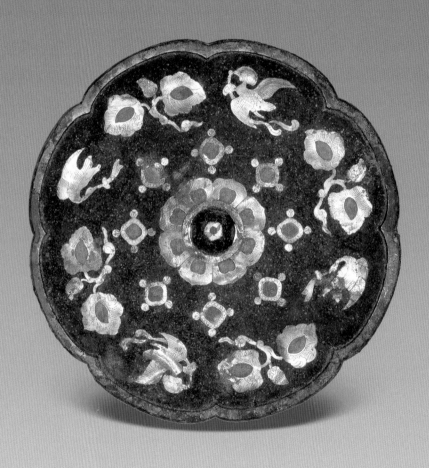

镶嵌螺钿花鸟葵花镜

唐

铜质

直径 24.5 厘米

八瓣葵花形。圆钮，莲瓣纹钮座。其外为一周团花纹。主纹分四组，每组饰鸾鸟衔绶、莲花荷叶纹各一。整个图案以绿松石为地，花鸟图案均以螺钿拼绘，纹饰线条刻画细致入微。

日本白鹤美术馆藏

Mallow Flower-shaped Mirror with Mother-of-Pearl Inlay

Tang Dynasty

Bronze

Diameter 24.5 cm

The mirror is in the shape of an eight-petaled mallow flower and has a hemispherical knob. The knob base is decorated with lotus petal designs, which are surrounded by a circle of flowers. There are four groups of principal motifs. Each one consists of a bird holding a ribbon in its beak and lotus leaves. The background is inlaid with turquoises while the motifs are mother-of-pearl inlays.

Preserved in Hakutsuru Fine Art Museum, Japan

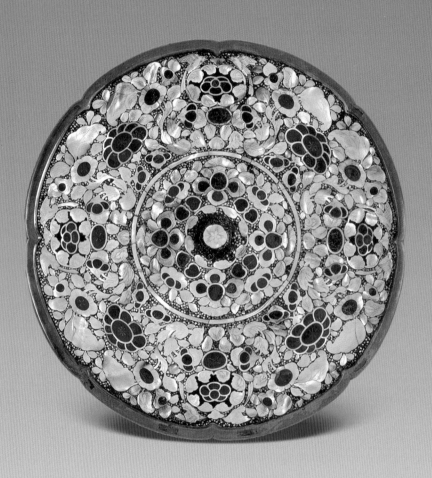

镶嵌螺钿莲花葵花镜

唐

铜质

直径 27.4 厘米

八瓣葵花形。圆钮,连珠纹钮座。内区饰花蕾、莲叶纹。外区为四朵大莲枝,中间为盛开的花瓣以及繁茂的枝叶、蔓生的花蕾。整个纹饰由玉石、青金石、贝壳、琥珀组成,色彩艳丽,具有极强的装饰性。

日本正仓院藏

Mallow Flower-shaped Mirror with Mother-of-Pearl Inlay

Tang Dynasty

Bronze

Diameter 27.4 cm

The mirror is in the shape of an eight-petaled mallow flower and has a hemispherical knob. The knob base is decorated with pearl designs, which are surrounded by flower buds and lotus leaves. The outer segment is decorated with patterns of flowers and leaves inlaid with colorful and decorative shells, jades, ambers and lapis lazulis.

Preserved in Shosoin, Japan

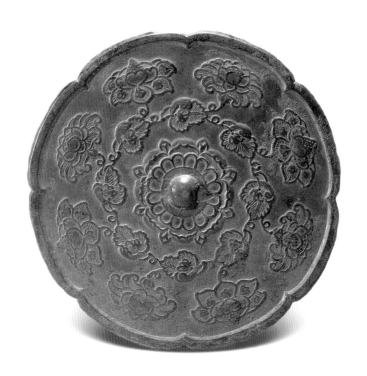

宝相花葵花镜

唐

铜质

直径 20.5 厘米

Mallow Flower-shaped Mirror with Rosette Designs

Tang dynasty

Bronze

Diameter 20.5 cm

八瓣葵花形。圆钮，莲花瓣钮座。钮外围枝
叶连接环绕成圈，并由枝蔓引出八朵宝相花
环绕其外。花分两种，或怒放，或初绽，均
为重瓣。陕西省西安市东郊出土。

陕西历史博物馆藏

The mirror is in the shape of an eight-petaled
mallow flower and has a hemispherical knob.
The knob base is decorated with lotus petals,
which are surrounded by branches and eight
rosette designs. The mirror was unearthed on
the eastern suburbs of Xi'an, Shaanxi Province.
Preserved in Shaanxi History Museum

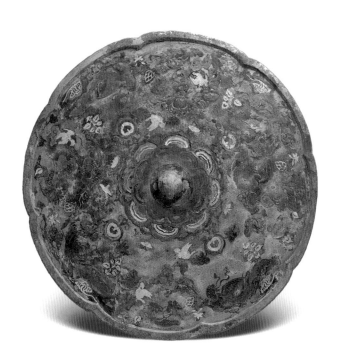

金银平脱羽人花鸟葵花镜

唐

铜质

直径 36.5 厘米

Lacquered Mallow Flower-shaped Mirror

Tang Dynasty

Bronze

Diameter 36.5 cm

八瓣葵花形。圆钮，重瓣莲花钮座。主纹为双羽人和双鸾展翅飞翔。间饰石榴花、蜂蝶、禽鸟和流云纹。均采用金银平脱法制作。河南省郑州市出土。

中国国家博物馆藏

The mirror is in the shape of an eight-petaled mallow flower and has a hemispherical knob. The knob base is decorated with double lotus petals. Its principal motifs consist of two winged people and two birds interspersed with pomegranate flowers, butterflies, birds, and clouds. All the designs are inlaid silver or gold sheets. The mirror was unearthed in Zhengzhou, Henan Province.

Preserved in National Museum of China

金银平脱鸾鸟衔绶镜

唐

铜质

直径 22.7 厘米

圆形。圆钮。其外为银饰莲叶纹，莲叶外饰一周金丝同心结纹。钮外围饰四只口衔绶带的金花鸾鸟，呈展翅飞翔状，鸾鸟间各饰一银饰菊花。近边缘处饰一周金丝同心结纹。陕西省西安市出土。

陕西历史博物馆藏

Lacquered Mirror Patterned with Birds

Tang Dynasty

Bronze

Diameter 22.7 cm

The mirror is round in shape. Its hemispherical knob is surrounded by patterns of lotus leaves enclosed by a ring of true lover's knots. The main motifs are four flying mythical birds with a ribbon in their beaks. Another ring of true lover's knots decorates the edge of the mirror. All the patterns are inlaid silver or gold sheets. The mirror was unearthed in Xi'an, Shaanxi Province.

Preserved in Shaanxi History Museum

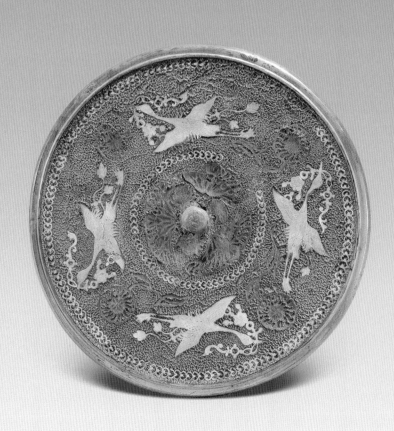

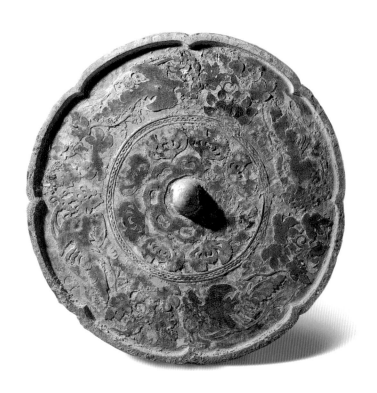

金银平脱花鸟葵花镜

唐

铜质

直径 30.5 厘米

八瓣葵花形，圆钮。镜背以金银片锤脱成四只展
翅环飞的鸾凤，并饰花鸟、飞蝶。河南省洛阳市
关林天宝九年（750）墓出土。

洛阳博物馆藏

Lacquered Mallow Flower-shaped Mirror Patterned with Birds and Flowers

Tang Dynasty

Bronze

Diameter 30.5 cm

The mirror is in the shape of an eight-petaled mallow flower and has a hemispherical knob. The main motifs are four flying phoenixes interspersed with birds, flowers, and butterflies, which are all inlaid silver or gold sheets. The mirror was unearthed from a tomb of Ninth-year Tianbao (750) Period in Guanlin, Luoyang City, Henan Province.

Preserved in Luoyang Museum

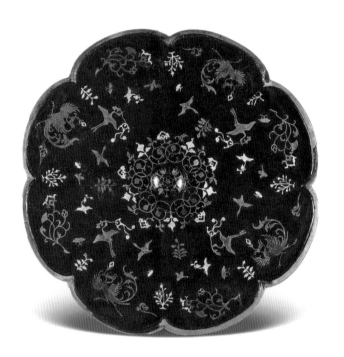

金银平脱花鸟葵花镜

唐

铜质

直径 28.5 厘米

Lacquered Mallow Flower-shaped Mirror Patterned with Birds and Flowers

Tang Dynasty

Bronze

Diameter 28.5 cm

八瓣葵花形。圆钮，饰宝相花。其外为缠绕的花枝，伸出十个花蕾。共有四组禽鸟环绕花丛飞翔，每组有大小不同的六只飞鸟。八葵瓣各有一只衔花鸾鸟和一株花枝。此镜纹饰用金银平脱方法制作，显示了一派鸟语花香的景象。

日本正仓院藏

The mirror is in the shape of an eight-petaled mallow flower. Its knob, hemispherical in shape, is decorated with rosette designs. Branches with ten flower buds surround the knob. Four groups of birds are flying amid the flowers with six birds of various size in each group. Along the edge of the mirror back, there are eight groups of mallow flower patterns with one bird holding a flower in its beak and one blooming bough in each pattern. All the patterns are inlaid silver or gold sheets.

Preserved in Shosoin, Japan

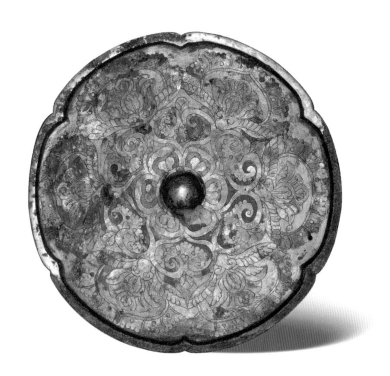

金银平脱葵花镜

唐

铜质

直径 19 厘米

Lacquered Mallow Flower-shaped Mirror

Tang Dynasty

Bronze

Diameter 19 cm

六瓣葵花形。圆钮，六瓣花形钮座，高平缘。

整体纹饰由圆形银片镂雕錾刻三层宝相花纹，

一层六重花瓣组成花形钮座，二层花瓣间伸出

六个含苞欲放的花蕾，花蕾外饰两片叶片托起

盛开的宝相花六朵。此镜纹饰华美，工艺独特，

漆地虽大部脱落，仍不失为一件精美的工艺品。

1955 年陕西省长安县（今长安区）韦曲出土。

中国国家博物馆藏

The mirror is in the shape of a six-petaled mallow flower and has a hemispherical knob. Its base is decorated with a flower of six petals. The main motifs consist of three rings of rosette designs. The innermost ring of six petals form the floral knob base. The middle ring is made up of six blooming buds. The outermost part is six rosettes supported by two leaves. All the designs are inlaid silver or gold sheets. Although most part of the lacquer has fallen off, the mirror is still a delicate piece of artwork for its gorgeous patterns and unique craftmanship. This artifact was unearthed at Weiqu of Chang'an County(now Chang'an District), Shaanxi Province.

Preserved in National Museum of China

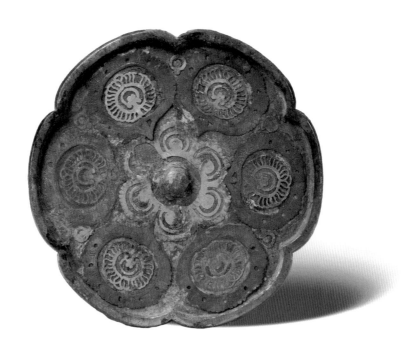

金银平脱镜

唐

铜质

直径 19 厘米

Lacquered Mirror

Tang Dynasty

Bronze

Diameter 19 cm

六瓣葵花形。圆钮。钮周围饰金片六出重瓣纹，每瓣为三重，其中一瓣残失二重。其外为六个银片心形纹中套金片宝相纹。心形纹之间缀金片瓣纹现存五枚。

济南市博物馆藏

The mirror is in the shape of a six-petaled mallow flower. Its hemispherical knob is surrounded by six patterns of triple petals. In the outer segment there are the principal motifs, six gold-sheet rosette designs enclosed by heart-shaped patterns in silver sheets. Only five rosette designs are left.

Preserved in Jinan Museum

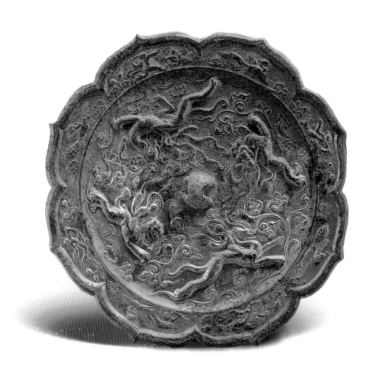

仙人骑兽菱花镜

唐

铜质

直径 25.5 厘米

Linghua-shaped Mirror Patterned with Immortals

Tang Dynasty

Bronze

Diameter 25.5 cm

八瓣菱花形。桥形钮。内区纹饰为四仙人骑
瑞兽呈奔驰状。仙人头顶光环，翱于天际，
隙间饰折枝花和流云。外区菱花瓣内饰鸟雀、
仙人，间饰以折枝花。1972 年陕西省西安市
郭家滩出土。

陕西历史博物馆藏

The mirror is in the shape of a linghua flower
with eight petals. Its knob is bridge-shaped.
The main motifs are four immortals riding on
supernatural animals with a halo around their
heads, which are interspersed with clouds and
flowers. Around the main motifs are patterns of
birds, flying fairies and flowers. This mirror was
unearthed at Guojiatan site of Xi'an, Shaanxi
Province, in 1972.

Preserved in Shaanxi History Museum

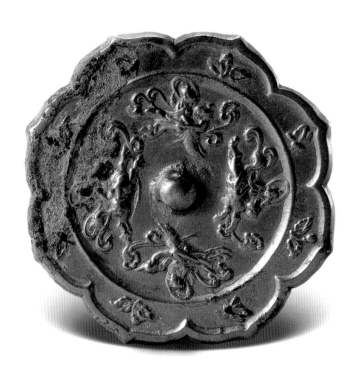

仙人骑兽菱花镜

唐

铜质

直径 11.5 厘米

Linghua-shaped Mirror Patterned with Immortals

Tang Dynasty

Bronze

Diameter 11.5 cm

八瓣菱花形。圆钮。内区饰四仙人各骑凤鸟
或神兽，外区饰四组飞蝶和折枝花。1983 年
陕西省凤翔棉纺厂出土。

陕西省考古研究院藏

The mirror is in the shape of a linghua flower
with eight petals and has a hemispherical knob.
The main motifs are four immortals riding on
supernatural animals, which are surrounded by
four groups of butterflies and plucked branches.
The mirror was excavated at Fengxiang Cotton
Mill, Shaanxi Province, in 1983.
Preserved in Shaanxi Provincial Institute of
Archaeology

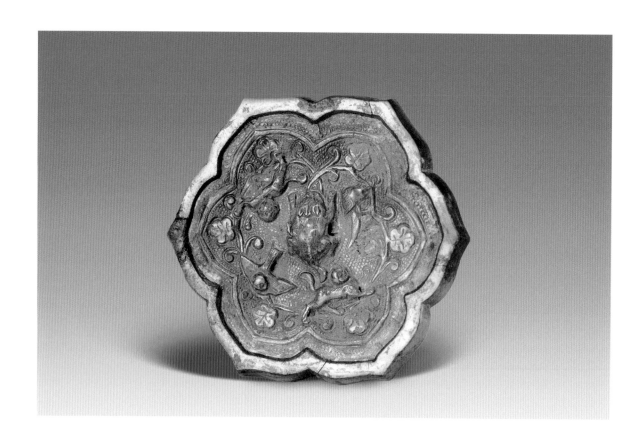

银背鎏金鸟兽菱花镜

唐

铜质

直径 11.2 厘米

Gilt Linghua-shaped Mirror Patterned with Birds and Beasts

Tang Dynasty

Bronze

Diameter 11.2 cm

六瓣菱花形。蟾蜍钮。银背鎏金。主题纹饰
为鸟兽及缠枝花，鸟兽对称排列。1992 年
陕西省西安市东郊出土。

陕西省考古研究院藏

The mirror is in the shape of a linghua flower
with six petals. Its knob is shaped like a toad
and its back is gilt silver. The main motifs
are birds, beasts, and interlocking flower
patterns, which are symmetrically arranged.
The mirror was unearthed on the eastern
suburbs of Xi'an, Shaanxi Province, in 1992.
Preserved in Shaanxi Provincial Institute of
Archaeology

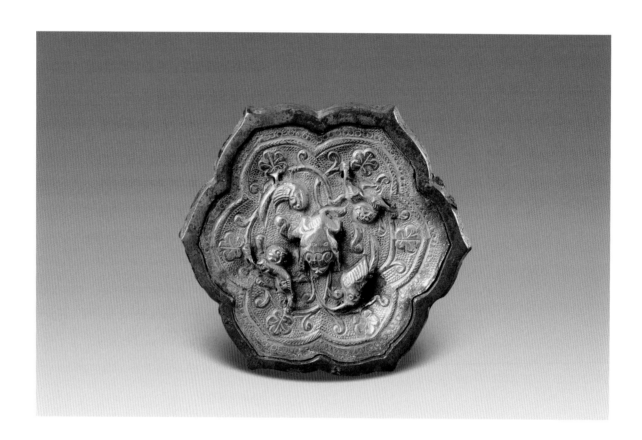

银背鎏金鸟兽菱花镜

唐

铜质

直径 11.2 厘米

Gilt Linghua-shaped Mirror Patterned with Birds and Beasts

Tang Dynasty

Bronze

Diameter 11.2 cm

六瓣菱花形。蟾蜍钮。银背鎏金。主题纹饰为鸟兽及缠枝花纹，以繁密的点纹为地纹。1993 年陕西省西安市东郊出土。

陕西省考古研究院藏

The mirror is in the shape of a linghua flower with six petals. Its knob is shaped like a toad and its back is gilt silver. The main motifs are birds, beasts, and interlocking flower patterns with pearl designs as the background. The mirror was unearthed on the eastern suburbs of Xi'an, Shaanxi Province, in 1993.

Preserved in Shaanxi Provincial Institute of Archaeology

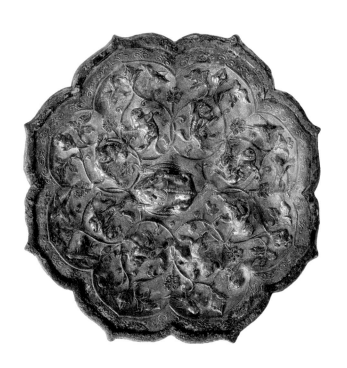

银背鎏金鸟兽菱花镜

唐

铜质

直径 19.3 厘米

Gilt Linghua-shaped Mirror Patterned with Birds and Beasts

Tang Dynasty

Bronze

Diameter 19.3 cm

八瓣菱花形。伏兽钮，连珠纹钮座。银背鎏金。由缠枝纹交错组成的八个圆弧内各饰一瑞兽，或回首，或奔走，姿态各异。在缠枝纹相接处饰石榴、荷花等，两侧间饰鸟禽、花叶。纹饰均以细密的圆圈纹为地。

日本白鹤美术馆藏

The mirror is in the shape of a linghua flower with eight petals. Its knob is shaped like a crouching animal. Its back is gilt silver. The interlocking flower patterns form eight circles with an auspicious animal with different postures in each. The principal motifs are interspersed with designs of pomegranates and lotuses, on both sides of which are birds, flowers and leaves. The background is designs of fine rings.

Preserved in Hakutsuru Fine Art Museum, Japan

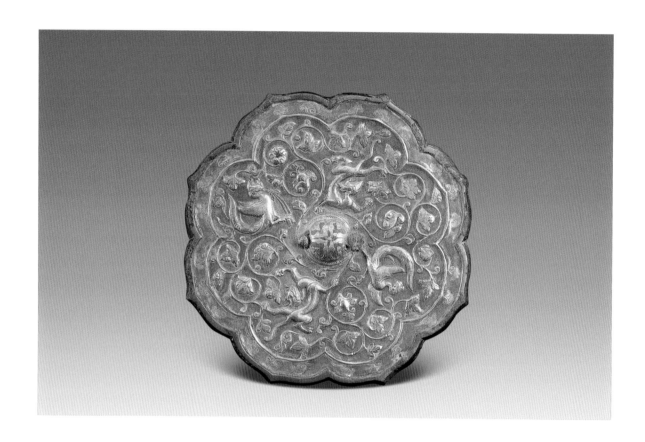

银背鎏金鸟兽菱花镜

唐

铜质

直径 21.2 厘米

Gilt Linghua-shaped Mirror Patterned with Birds and Beasts

Tang Dynasty

Bronze

Diameter 21.2 cm

八瓣菱花形。圆钮，连珠纹钮座。银背鎏金。

钮的周围饰两鸟两兽。两鸟展翅翘尾，一鸟

口衔绶带。两兽一爪屈伸，三爪舒展，体躯

弯曲，呈张牙舞爪状，兽与鸟之间饰折枝花。

外缘为云纹和花饰。整个纹饰均以细珠纹

为地。

日本千石唯司藏

The mirror is in the shape of a linghua flower with eight petals. Its hemispherical knob sits on the knob base decorated with the design of pearls. Its back is gilt silver. Two birds and two beasts surround the knob. The birds are spreading their wings and tails and one of them is holding a ribbon in its beak. The animals are bent over towards their back, waving one of their paws. The birds and beasts are interspersed with patterns of plucked branches. The edge of the mirror is decorated with clouds and flowers. Fine pearl designs are the background.

Preserved in Sengoku Tadashi Museum, Japan

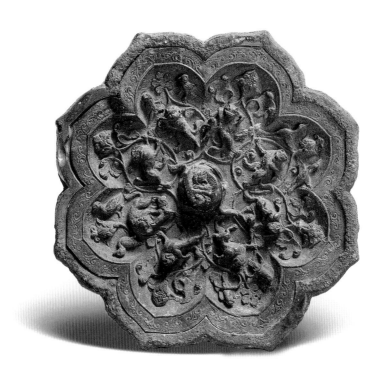

银背鸟兽菱花镜

唐

铜质

直径 15.8 厘米

Linghua-shaped Mirror Patterned with Birds and Beasts

Tang Dynasty

Bronze

Diameter 15.8 cm

八瓣菱花形。兽钮，呈头尾相拥状。镜心由缠枝花组成八个区域，内各有一只瑞兽，似狻猊。菱花瓣内饰石榴、花卉，并间隔饰以双雀，或栖于花枝，或展翅飞翔。此镜均以细珠纹为地。双兽钮镜较为稀见。陕西省西安市史家营出土。

陕西历史博物馆藏

The mirror is in the shape of a linghua flower with eight petals. The knob was made in the shape of two cuddling animals. The interlocking flowers divide the mirror back into eight segments with a lion in each. The main motifs are surrounded by patterns of pomegranates and flowers, which are interspersed with pairs of sparrows flying or resting on branches. Patterns of pearls are the background. The mirror was unearthed at Shijiaying site of Xi'an, Shaanxi Province.

Preserved in Shaanxi History Museum

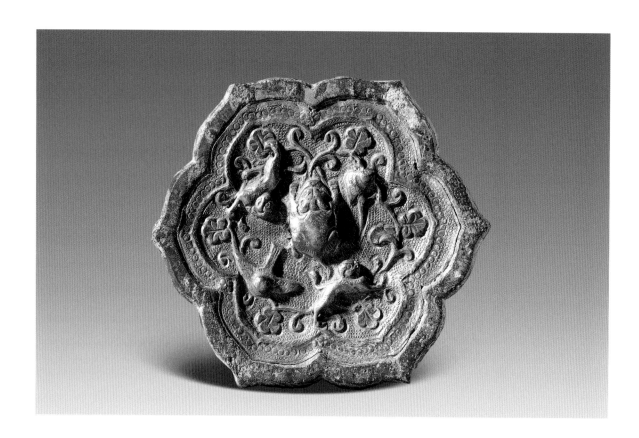

银背鸟兽菱花镜

唐

铜质

直径 6.2 厘米

Linghua-shaped Mirror Patterned with Birds and Beasts

Tang Dynasty

Bronze

Diameter 6.2 cm

六角菱花形。兽钮。镜背浮雕两雀、两瑞兽
与缠枝花相间环绕。此镜银地鎏金，以锤脱
工艺制成。河南省洛阳市老井村出土。

洛阳博物馆藏

The mirror is in the shape of a linghua flower
with six petals and has an animal-shaped knob.
Two beasts and two magpies comprise the
principal motifs which are interspersed with
interlocking flowers. The back of the mirror
is gilt. This artifact was excavated at Laojing
Village of Luoyang City, Henan Province.
Preserved in Luoyang Museum

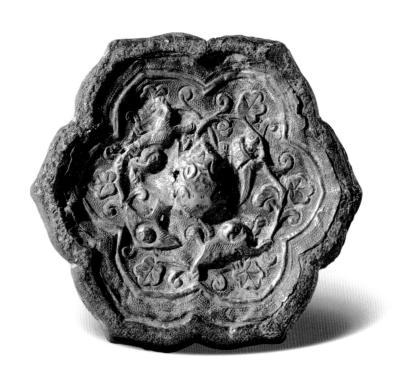

银背鸟兽菱花镜

唐

铜质

直径 5.9 厘米

Linghua-shaped Mirror Patterned with Birds and Beasts

Tang Dynasty

Bronze

Diameter 5.9 cm

六瓣菱花形。蛙钮，银背。镜心纹饰为对称
排列的两瑞兽和两雀。瑞兽呈奔跑状，一雀
展翅，一雀栖于枝头。河南省洛阳市出土。

洛阳博物馆藏

The mirror is in the shape of a linghua flower
with six petals and has a frog-shaped knob.
Two birds and two racing beasts arranged
symmetrically comprise the principal motifs.
The mirror was unearthed in Luoyang City,
Henan Province.

Preserved in Luoyang Museum

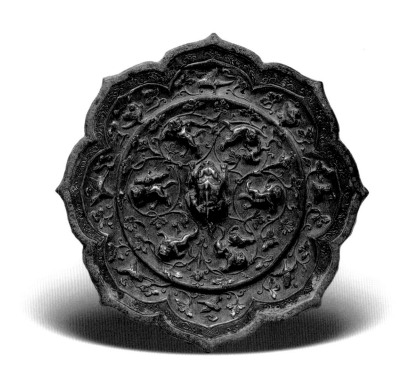

银背鸟兽菱花镜

唐

铜质

直径 21.5 厘米

Linghua-shaped Mirror Patterned with Birds and Beasts

Tang Dynasty

Bronze

Diameter 21.5 cm

八瓣菱花形。伏兽钮。银背。内区饰缠枝花纹，
枝叶间饰六只瑞兽。外区饰姿态各异的八只
雀鸟，间以花草纹。镜缘饰流云纹。1955 年
陕西省西安市出土。

陕西历史博物馆藏

The mirror is in the shape of a linghua flower
with eight petals. The knob is shaped like a
crouching animal. A raised ring divides the
main motifs into two segments. The inner
segment is decorated with interlocking branches
and flowers, which are interspersed with six
auspicious animals. In the outer segment there
are eight birds in various postures, which are
interspersed with flowers and grass. The edge
of the mirror is patterned with cloud designs.
This mirror was unearthed in Xi'an, Shaanxi
Province, in 1955.

Preserved in Shaanxi History Museum

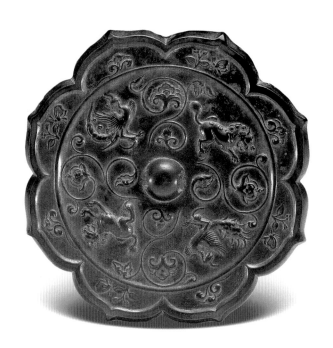

鸟兽菱花镜

唐

铜质

直径 15.6 厘米

Linghua-shaped Mirror Patterned with Birds and Beasts

Tang Dynasty

Bronze

Diameter 15.6 cm

八瓣菱花形。圆钮。内区饰枝蔓向两侧弯曲
的宝相花四枝，对称饰凤凰纹、瑞兽纹，凤
凰呈回首状，瑞兽张嘴翘尾。外区菱花瓣内
饰蝴蝶采花纹样。四川省平武县出土。

四川博物院藏

The mirror is shaped like a linghua flower with
eight petals and has a hemispherical knob. A
raised ring divides the main motifs into two
segments. The inner segment is decorated with
two phoenixes, two auspicious animals, and
four rosettes. There are butterflies and flowers
in the outer segment. The mirror was unearthed
in Pingwu County, Sichuan Province.
Preserved in Sichuan Museum

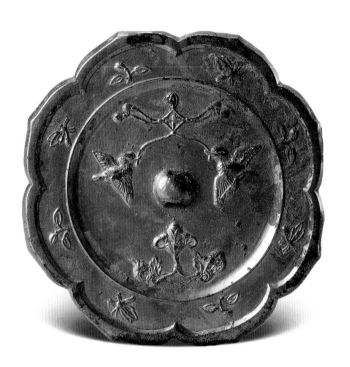

飞鸟菱花镜

唐

铜质

直径 14.5 厘米

Linghua-shaped Mirror Patterned with Flying Birds

Tang Dynasty

Bronze

Diameter 14.5 cm

八瓣菱花形。圆钮。上部饰灯笼形图案和菱形图案，上下相连，菱形图案两侧饰绶带飘扬，下角亦饰两条绶带，两鸟各衔一条呈飞翔状；下部饰荷花一组。八个葵瓣间饰飞蝶及折枝花。1983年陕西省凤翔县棉纺厂出土。

陕西省考古研究院藏

The mirror is shaped like a linghua flower with eight petals and has a hemispherical shape. The main motifs are divided into two segments. In the upper segment there are one group of lantern-shaped patterns and one group of diamond-shaped patterns linked with each other. On each side of the latter patterns, there is a waving ribbon. The middle lower corner of the diamond is tied with a ribbon held in the beak of a flying bird on each side. Underneath there is a group of a lotus and leaves. The edge of the mirror is decorated with butterflies and flowers. The mirror was unearthed at Fengxiang Cotton Mill, Shaanxi Province, in 1983.

Preserved in Shaanxi Provincial Institute of Archaeology

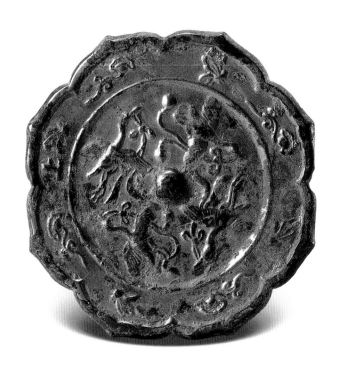

飞鸟菱花镜

唐

铜质

直径 12.6 厘米

Linghua-shaped Mirror Patterned with Flying Birds

Tang Dynasty

Bronze

Diameter 12.6 cm

八瓣菱花形。圆钮。内区饰四只口衔绶带的
鸿雁，呈飞翔状；外区饰四组如意云纹及花
草。1991年陕西省西安市东郊出土。

陕西省考古研究院藏

The mirror is shaped like a linghua flower of
eight petals and has a hemispherical knob. The
main motifs are divided into two segments.
There are four flying wild geese with ribbons
in their beaks in the inner segment. The outer
segment is decorated with patterns of clouds
and flowers. This mirror was unearthed on the
eastern suburbs of Xi'an, Shaanxi Province, in
1991.
Preserved in Shaanxi Provincial Institute of
Archaeology

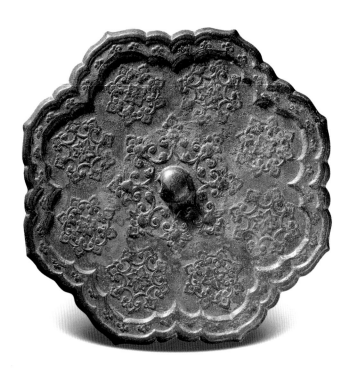

宝相花菱花镜

唐

铜质

直径 23.3 厘米

Linghua-shaped Mirror Patterned with Rosette Designs

Tang Dynasty

Bronze

Diameter 23.3 cm

八瓣菱花形，花瓣纹钮座。八角顶端向外放
射同形的花叶形纹。八朵宝相花环绕钮座，
宝相花为八瓣形，四瓣花形蕊。外缘均匀地
排列四十朵小花。此镜纹饰规整，清新雅致。

中国国家博物馆藏

The mirror is shaped like a linghua flower with
eight petals. The knob is hemispherical with
a knob base in the shape of an eight-petaled
flower. The main motifs are eight patterns of
rosettes with each having eight petals. The edge
of the mirror is evenly decorated with forty
little flowers. The patterns are well structured
and elegant.

Preserved in National Museum of China

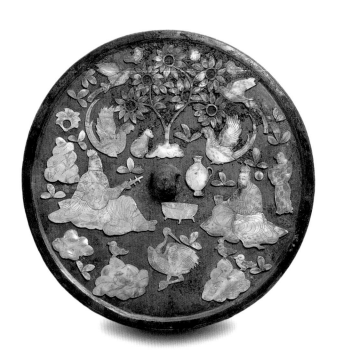

镶嵌螺钿人物花鸟镜

唐

铜质

直径 23.9 厘米

Mirror with Mother-of-pearl Inlay

Tang Dynasty

Bronze

Diameter 23.9 cm

圆形。圆钮，纹饰用螺钿镶嵌成一幅图画。画中两老翁坐于树前，左侧一人弹阮，右侧一人持杯欲饮，前置一壶一樽，后有一侍女捧物侍立。树下蹲坐一犬，两侧鹦鹉展翅。树梢上饰对称四鸟，小鸟立于枝头，大鸟振翅于树梢。下有一只鹭鸶和三只小鸟，其间点缀草石落叶。嵌螺钿青铜镜是唐代著名的工艺珍品。1955 年河南省洛阳市出土。

中国国家博物馆藏

This round mirror has a hemispherical knob. On the back of the mirror, there is a scene of two old men sitting in front of a tree. The one on the left is playing an stringed musical instrument while the other is holding a cup about to drink. A maid is standing behind him. There are also birds, a dog, an egret, rocks, flowers and grass in this scene. All the motifs are mother-of-pearl inlays. Bronze mirrors with mother-of-pearl inlay were precious pieces of artwork in the Tang Dynasty. The mirror was unearthed in Luoyang, Henan Province, in 1955.

Preserved in National Museum of China

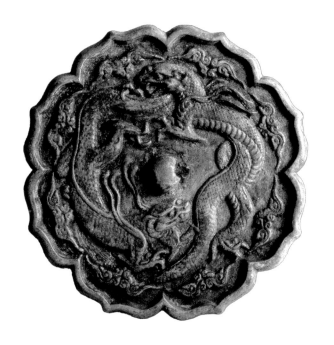

双龙镜

唐

铜质

直径 19.5 厘米

Mirror of Double Dragons

Tang Dynasty

Bronze

Diameter 19.5 cm

八瓣菱花形。圆钮，钮外二龙环绕，刻画清晰。每瓣菱花边下均配置云纹，用以衬托龙腾祥云的气势。传出南京南郊。

南京博物院藏

The mirror is shaped like a linghua flower with eight petals. The knob, hemispherical in shape, is surrounded by two dragons. The edge of the mirror is decorated with cloud patterns which were intended to foreground the atmosphere of dragons speeding on auspicious clouds. It is believed that the mirror was unearthed on the southern suburbs of Nanjing City.

Preserved in Nanjing Museum

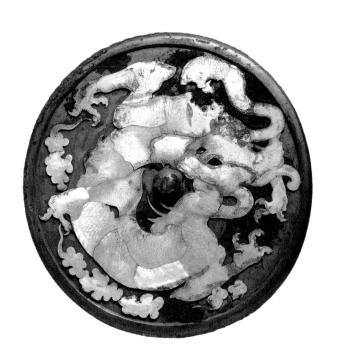

镶嵌螺钿云龙纹镜

唐

铜质

直径 22 厘米

Mother-of-pearl Inlay Mirror with Clouds and Dragon Patterned

Tang Dynasty

Bronze

Diameter 22 cm

圆形。圆钮。主题纹饰为一用镶嵌螺钿工艺拼绘的龙，龙首衔钮，体躯弯曲而上，前肢一伸一曲，二后肢与龙首相交。龙周围饰流云纹，使之有腾云驾雾之感。背鳍、腹甲、鳞甲、肘毛刻画精细。河南省陕县后川出土。

中国国家博物馆藏

This round mirror has a hemispherical knob. Its back is decorated with a dragon looking back over its shoulders with the knob in its mouth. The body of the dragon was engraved with fineness. Clouds surround the dragon. All the patterns are mother-of-pearl inlays. The mirror was unearthed in Houchuan of Shanxian County, Henan Province.

Preserved in National Museum of China

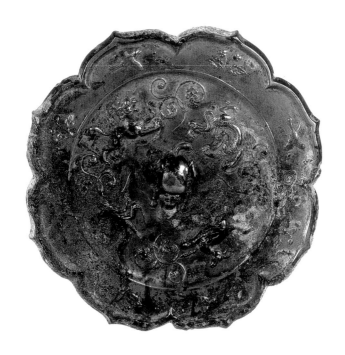

鸢鸟瑞兽铜镜

唐

铜质

直径 22.2 厘米

Bronze Mirror Patterned with Birds and Beasts

Tang Dynasty

Bronze

Diameter 22.2 cm

八瓣菱花形。兽形钮。钮外四周以高浮雕相间配置鸾凤、麒麟及似狐似狼的瑞兽四只。麒麟张牙舞爪，鸾凤展翅欲飞，瑞兽绕钮奔驰，表态各异栩栩如生；鸾兽之间饰以卷草；外缘是排列有序的飞禽、蜂蝶和花枝。此镜厚重，表面包浆呈银白色，有别一般唐镜的古铜色或黑漆色，为扬州本土铸造。江苏省高邮市出土。

高邮市博物馆藏

The mirror is in the shape of a linghua flower with eight petals and has an animal-shaped knob. A phoenix, a dragon, a kylin, and another nameless animal in high relief comprise the principal motifs, which are separated by a raised ring from designs of flying birds, butterflies, branches and flowers. The mirror, thick and heavy, has a silvery wrapped slurry on its surface, which is different from bronze or lacquer color of ordinary mirrors in the Tang Dynasty. The mirror was made in Yangzhou City and unearthed in Gaoyou City, Jiangsu Province.

Preserved in Gaoyou Museum

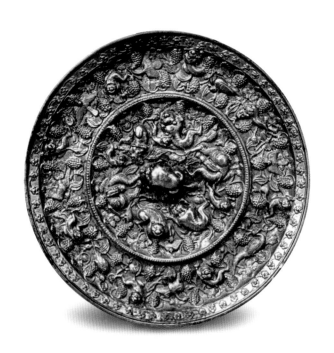

瑞兽葡萄镜

唐

铜质

直径 21.6 厘米

Mirror Patterned with Auspicious Animals and Grapes

Tang Dynasty

Bronze

Diameter 21.6 cm

圆形。伏兽钮。内外区均表现缠枝葡萄与珍禽异兽的形象，其中内区分布六只动态各异的瑞兽；外区则为十六只禽鸟与瑞兽相间，在葡萄枝叶间隐现。

山西博物院藏

The round mirror has a knob in the shape of a crouching animal. A raised ring divides the principal motifs into two segments, both of which are decorated with exotic animals and grapes. The six animals in the inner segment are all in various postures. In the outer segment there are sixteen birds and auspicious animals arranged alternately and separated by grape tree branches.

Preserved in Shanxi Museum

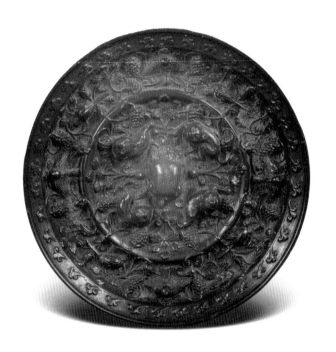

瑞兽葡萄镜

唐

铜质

直径 12.8 厘米

Mirror Patterned with Auspicious Animals and Grapes

Tang Dynasty

Bronze

Diameter 12.8 cm

圆形。伏兽钮。内区有葡萄枝蔓叶实缠绕，
四瑞兽呈攀援状；外区满饰叶实累累的葡萄
枝蔓，八只禽鸟穿插其间，或展翅欲飞，或
栖息枝上。流云纹缘。

南京市博物馆藏

The round mirror has a knob in the shape of
a crouching animal. A raised ring divides the
principal motifs into two segments. The inner
segment is decorated with four auspicious
animals climbing the grapes tree branches,
while the outer segment is filled with grapes
and branches interspersed with eight flying or
resting birds. The edge of the mirror is patterned
with clouds.

Preserved in Nanjing Municipal Museum

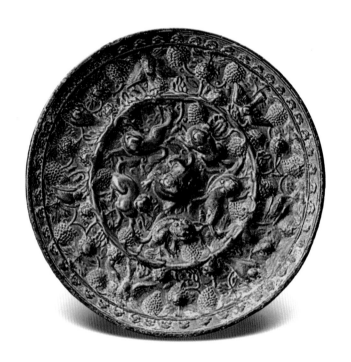

禽兽葡萄镜

唐

铜质

直径 14.4 厘米

Mirror Patterned with Auspicious Animals and Grapes

Tang Dynasty

Bronze

Diameter 14.4 cm

圆形。兽钮。镜背一周枝蔓状凸弦纹分为内外
两区，内区饰戏水海兽，外区环绕禽鸟，葡萄
枝蔓间饰内外禽兽纹间。花云纹窄外缘。

山西博物院藏

The round mirror has a knob in the shape of
a crouching animal. A raised ring of branches
divides the principal motifs into two segments.
The inner segment is decorated with sea animals
playing in the water while the outer segment is
decorated with flying birds. They are interspersed
with grape and vine designs. The narrow edge of
the mirror is patterned with clouds.

Preserved in Shanxi Museum

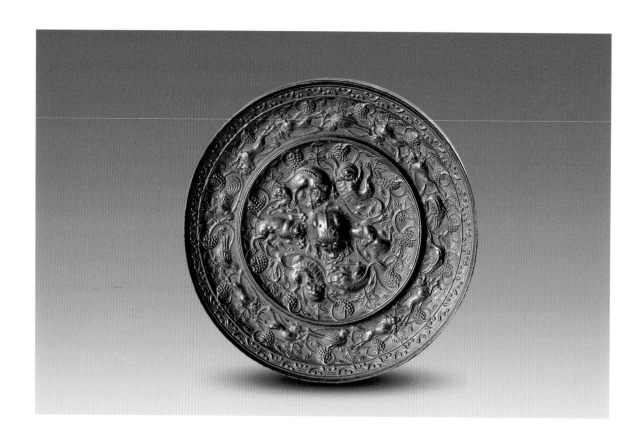

狻猊葡萄镜

唐

铜质

直径 15.2 厘米

Mirror Patterned with Lions and Grapes

Tang Dynasty

Bronze

Diameter 15.2 cm

圆形。兽钮。内区饰狻猊葡萄纹，外区饰凤鸟和异兽，边缘饰葡萄纹。纹饰皆采用高浮雕手法制作，工艺精良。1952 年陕西省西安市出土。

陕西历史博物馆藏

The round mirror has an animal-shaped knob. A raised ring of branches divides the principal motifs into two segments. The inner segment is decorated with lions and grape patterns while the outer segment has phoenixes and exotic animals. The edge of the mirror is patterned with grapes. All the patterns are in high relief, which shows exquisite craftmanship. The mirror was unearthed in Xi'an, Shaanxi Province, in 1952.

Preserved in Shaanxi History Museum

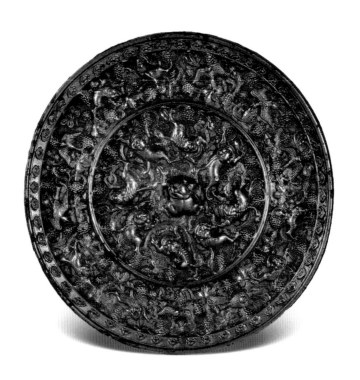

狻猊葡萄镜

唐

铜质

直径 23.9 厘米

Mirror Patterned with Lions and Grapes

Tang Dynasty

Bronze

Diameter 23.9 cm

圆形。狻猊钮。内区有八只狻猊姿态各异，隙间饰葡萄纹。外区有飞禽七只，狻猊三对，上下饰葡萄及枝叶纹。镜缘饰重瓣花。此镜纹饰交错，极其精奇富丽。

上海博物馆藏

The round mirror has a lion-shaped knob. A raised ring of branches divides the principal motifs into two segments. The inner segment is decorated with eight lions in various postures interspersed with grapes and branches, while the outer segment has three pairs of lions and seven birds separated by grapes and branches. The edge of the mirror is patterned with flowers. The patterns are interlocked in a gorgeous and complex manner.

Preserved in Shanghai Museum

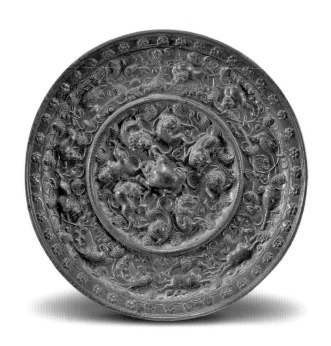

狻猊葡萄镜

唐

铜质

直径 24.7 厘米

Mirror Patterned with Lions and Grapes

Tang Dynasty

Bronze

Diameter 24.7 cm

圆形。兽钮，圆钮座。主题纹饰为高浮雕狻猊葡萄纹，间以禽、兽等纹饰。边缘凸起，颇显厚重。河南省宜阳县出土。

洛阳博物馆藏

The round mirror has an animal-shaped knob. The principal motifs are lions and grapes which are interspersed with birds and animals. The edge is raised, which makes the mirror look very thick and heavy. The mirror was unearthed in Yiyang County, Henan Province.
Preserved in Luoyang Museum

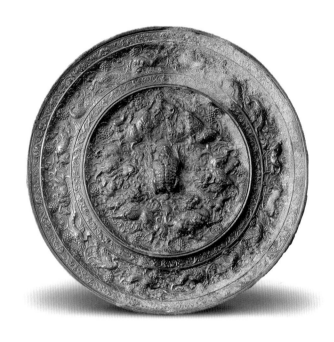

狻猊葡萄镜

唐

铜质

直径 17.1 厘米

Mirror Patterned with Lions and Grapes

Tang Dynasty

Bronze

Diameter 17.1 cm

圆形。狻猊钮。内区饰狻猊六只，或奔跑，或蹲坐，或安卧，或匍匐，间饰以缠枝花。外区置狻猊、飞雀、缠枝葡萄一周。镜缘饰缠枝纹。

日本千石唯司藏

The round mirror has a knob in the shape of a lion. A raised ring of branches divides the principal motifs into two segments. The inner segment is decorated with six lions with various postures , such as running, squating, sitting and creeping, among the lions, there also interspersed with interlocking flowers. The outer segment is filled with grapes, branches, lions and flying birds. The edge of the mirror is patterned with flowers.

Preserved in Sengoku Tadashi Museum, Japan

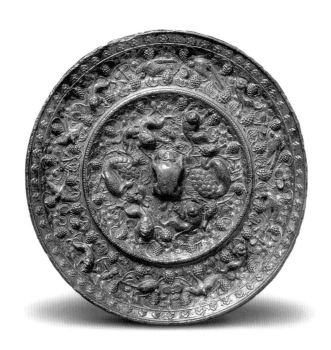

狻猊葡萄镜

唐

铜质

直径 21 厘米

Mirror Patterned with Lions and Grapes

Tang Dynasty

Bronze

Diameter 21 cm

圆形。伏兽钮。内区饰以狻猊和缠枝葡萄纹，

外区为鸟雀、蝴蝶、狻猊配以缠枝葡萄，缘

饰重瓣花纹一周。1958 年河南省陕县出土。

中国国家博物馆藏

The round mirror has a knob in the shape of a crouching animal. A raised ring of branches divides the principal motifs into two segments. The inner segment is decorated with lions, grapes and interlocking branches, while the outer segment is filled with birds, butterflies and lions separated by grape designs. The edge of the mirror is patterned with flowers. The mirror was unearthed in Shanxian, Henan Province, in 1958.

Preserved in National Museum of China

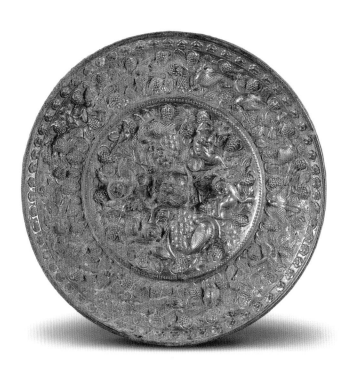

狻猊孔雀葡萄镜

唐

铜质

直径 20 厘米

Mirror Patterned with Lions, a Peacock and Grapes

Tang Dynasty

Bronze

Diameter 20 cm

圆形。蟠龙钮，龙首回顾。内区饰一开屏孔

雀，四只狻猊伏地昂首。间杂以蔓枝葡萄。

外区为姿态各异的喜鹊十二只，间杂以葡萄、

蜻蜓、蝴蝶等，纹饰形象生动，错落有致，

繁密华丽。

上海博物馆藏

The round mirror has a knob in the shape of a
coiled dragon. A raised ring of branches divides
the principal motifs into two segments. The
inner segment is decorated with four crouching
lions and a peacock showing its tail feathers. In
the outer segment there are twelve magpies with
different postures interspersed with designs of
butterflies, dragonflies and grapes. The patterns
are lively, gorgeous and well arranged.
Preserved in Shanghai Museum

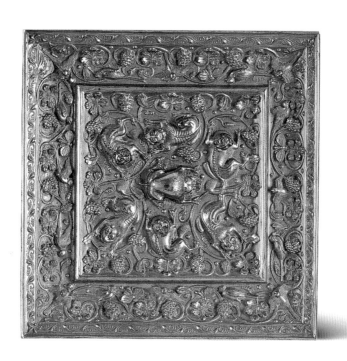

狻猊葡萄方镜

唐

铜质

边长 17.1 厘米

Square Mirror Patterned with Lions and Grapes

Tang Dynasty

Bronze

Side Length 17.1 cm

方形。伏兽钮。内区以钮为中心置六狻猊，间饰以葡萄缠枝纹。外区饰鸟雀、蝴蝶，配以葡萄缠枝纹。镜缘饰缠枝纹。此镜纹饰采用高浮雕技法制作，极为精美。

日本正仓院藏

The mirror is square and its knob resembles a crouching animal. A raised square divides the principal motifs into two segments. The inner segment is decorated with six lions interspersed with grapes and branches. In the outer segment there are birds and butterflies separated by grapes and interlocking branches. The edge of the mirror is patterned with interlocking branches. The exquisite patterns are all in high relief.

Preserved in Shosoin, Japan

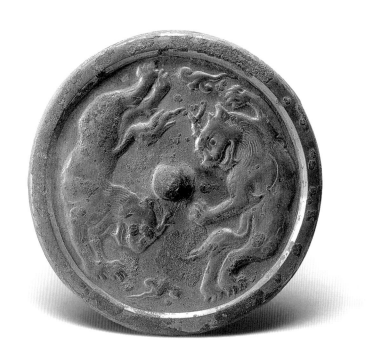

双狮纹镜

唐

铜质

直径 18.5 厘米

Mirror Patterned with Two Lions

Tang Dynasty

Bronze

Diameter 18.5 m

圆形。圆钮。钮外圈饰双狮，环绕镜钮，呈
追逐嬉戏状。镜背装饰具浮雕效果。陕西省
西安市东郊出土。

陕西历史博物馆藏

The round mirror has a hemispherical knob. Two
lions are playing around the knob. The patterns
on the back of the mirror are in relief. The mirror
was excavated on the eastern suburbs of Xi'an,
Shaanxi Province.

Preserved in Shaanxi History Museum

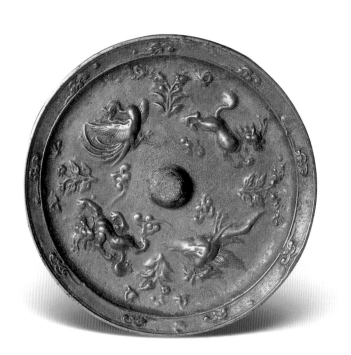

鸟兽纹镜

唐

铜质

直径 18.6 厘米

Mirror Patterned with Birds and Beasts

Tang Dynasty

Bronze

Diameter 18.6 m

圆形。圆钮。主题纹饰为对称分布的神兽、凤鸟，间饰四株花草及云纹。边缘饰云纹一周。1983 年陕西省西安市东郊出土。

陕西省考古研究院藏

The round mirror has a hemispherical knob. Around the knob there are two birds and two supernatural animals interspersed with designs of clouds, flowers and grass. The edge of the mirror is decorated with floating clouds. The mirror was excavated on the eastern suburbs of Xi'an, Shaanxi Province, in 1983.

Preserved in Shaanxi Provincial Institute of Archaeology

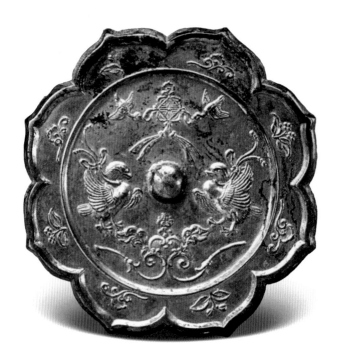

花鸟纹镜

唐

铜质

直径 17 厘米

Mirror Patterned with Birds and Flowers

Tang Dynasty

Bronze

Diameter 17 cm

八瓣菱花形。圆钮。内区钮两侧饰双鸾，上方饰双雀衔同心结，下饰盛开的花朵；外区环饰朵花图案。窄素凸缘。

山西博物院藏

The mirror is made in the shape of a linghua flower with eight petals. In the inner region there are two phoenixes standing on each side of the knob. Above the knob two sparrows are holding a ribbon in their beaks. Beneath the knob flowers are in full bloom. The outer region is decorated with flower motifs. Its convex rim is narrow and plain.

Preserved in Shanxi Museum

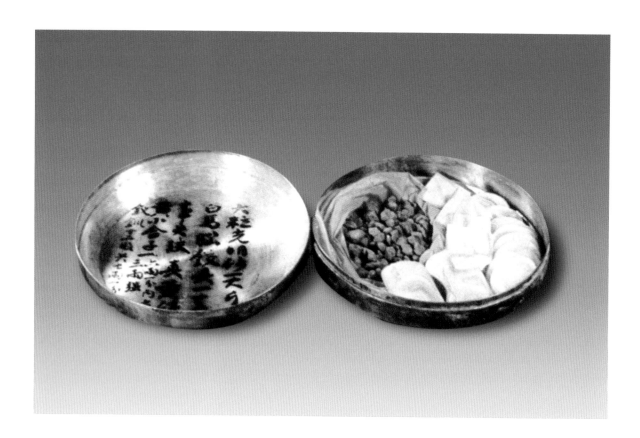

银药盒

唐

银质

口径 16.7 厘米，高 4.6 厘米

Silver Medicine Box

Tang Dynasty

Silver

Mouth Diameter 16.7 cm/ Height 4.6 cm

扁圆形。有盖。盖内有墨书"大粒光明砂一大斤，白玛瑙铰具一十五事，口玦真黄，纯黄小盒"等45字。盒内盛光明砂、白玛瑙等炼丹原料。1970年西安市何家村出土。

陕西历史博物馆藏

The oblate medicine box has a lid with 45 inscriptions on its inner surface indicating the materials in it and their weight. This box contains raw materials for alchemy including cinnabar and white agate. The box was unearthed at Hejiacun site, Xi'an City, in 1970.

Preserved in Shaanxi History Museum

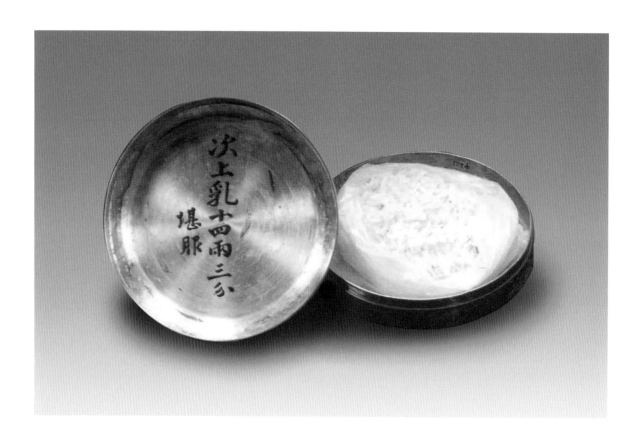

银药盒

唐

银质

口径 16.7 厘米，高 4.6 厘米

Silver Medicine Box

Tang Dynasty

Silver

Mouth Diameter 16.7 cm/ Height 4.6 cm

扁圆形，有盖，盖内有墨书"次上乳十四两三分，堪服"字样。1970 年陕西省西安市何家村出土。

陕西历史博物馆藏

The box is oblate. On the inner surface of its lid, there are inscriptions written in black ink about what was buried. The box was unearthed at Hejiacun site, Xi'an City, Shaanxi Province in 1970.

Preserved in Shaanxi History Museum

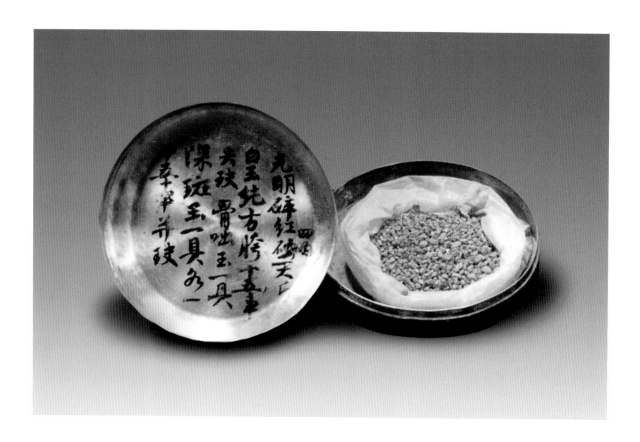

银药盒

唐

银质

口径 16.7 厘米，高 4.6 厘米

Silver Medicine Box

Tang Dynasty

Silver

Mouth Diameter 16.7cm/ Height 4.6 cm

扁圆形。有盖，盖内有墨书"四为光明碎红砂一大斤，白玉纯方胯十五事，尖玦骨咄玉一具，深斑玉一具，各一十五事并玦"。盒内盛光明砂，为炼丹原料。1970 年陕西省西安市何家村出土。

陕西历史博物馆藏

The box is oblate. On the inner surface of its lid there are inscriptions written in black ink about what was buried. The box contains cinnabar, a raw material for alchemy. The box was unearthed at Hejiacun site, Xi'an City, Shaanxi Province in 1970.

Preserved in Shaanxi History Museum

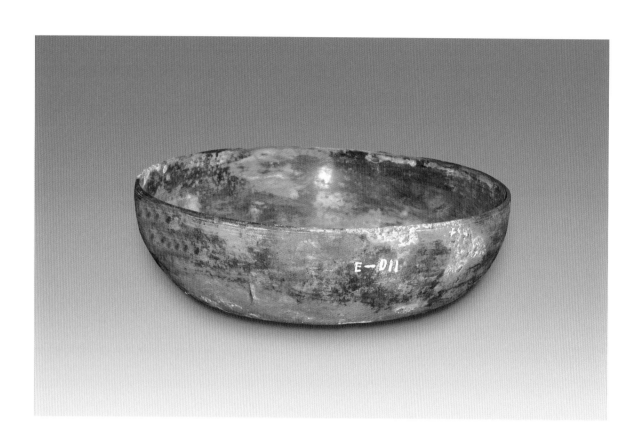

铜锅

唐

铜质

口径 23.2 厘米，底径 15 厘米，通高 7.6 厘米，
重 510 克

敞口，圆腹，无纹饰。底有修补。为炊器。陕西
省西安市鄠邑区征集。

陕西医史博物馆藏

Bronze Pot

Tang Dynasty

Bronze

Mouth Diameter 23.2 cm/ Bottom Diameter 15 cm/
Height 7.6 cm/ Weight 510 g

The cooking pot has a flared orifice and a round
belly. It has been repaired in its bottom. The artifact
was collected in Hu County, Xi'an City, Shaanxi
Province.

Preserved in Shaanxi Museum of Medical History

铜盆

唐

铜质

口径 22.5 厘米，底径 18 厘米，通高 13 厘米，
重 1000 克

平沿，圆腹，平底。有修补。为盛贮器。陕西省
西安市鄠邑区征集。

陕西医史博物馆藏

Bronze Basin

Tang Dynasty

Bronze

Mouth Diameter 22.5 cm/ Bottom Diameter 18 cm/
Height 13 cm/ Weight 1, 000 g

The basin has a flat rim, a round belly, and a flat
bottom. It has been repaired. The basin was used
for storage. It was collected in Huyi County, Xi'an
City, Shaanxi Province.

Preserved in Shaanxi Museum of Medical History

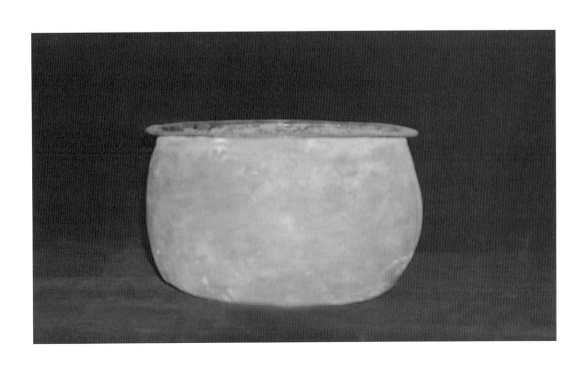

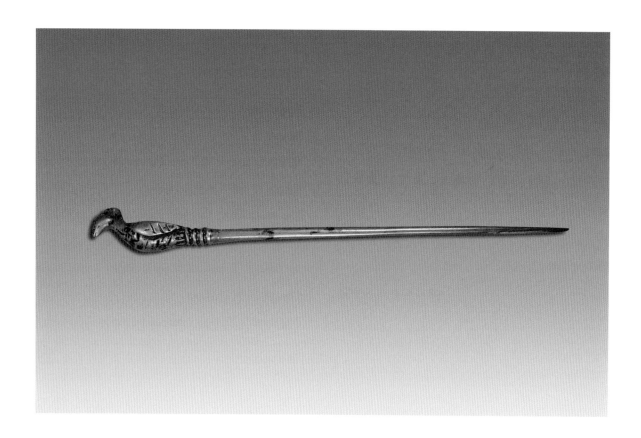

扁鹊纹银质针

唐

银质

长 13 厘米，径 3 厘米

Silver Needle with Bian Que Patterns

Tang Dynasty

Silver

Length 13 cm/ Diameter 3 cm

唐代早期医用器具。针形，上端有扁鹊图腾。
由于扁鹊对于中医发展的影响，故从战国后
期开始，很多医用工具，特别是针具经常出
现扁鹊饰物及图腾。

张雅宗藏

The artifact, a medical device in the early Tang
Dynasty, is shaped like a needle with its top
decorated with the totem of Bian Que, a famous
doctor in ancient China. After late Warring State
Period, many medical tools, especially needles,
were decorated with patterns and totem of
Bian Que because of his great influence on the
development of Traditional Chinese Medicine.
Collected by Zhang Yazong

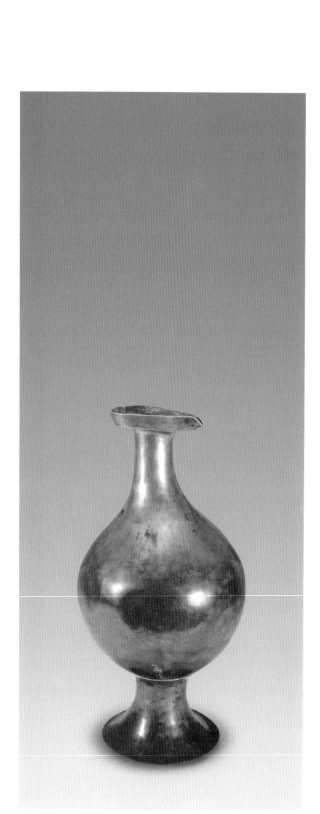

银执壶

唐

银质

腹径 13.5 厘米，通高 36.5 厘米

Silver Ewer

Tang Dynasty

Silver

Belly Diameter 13.5 cm/ Height 36.5 cm

带流式盘口，细长颈，溜肩，长圆腹，喇叭形
高圈足。口、腹间原有一执柄，已缺。器物造
型修长优美，具有浓郁的波斯萨珊王朝风格。

河北博物院藏

This ewer has a dish-shaped mouth with a spout.
Its neck is long and narrow, but its belly is
relatively long and round. The base is high and
looks like a trumpet. There used to be a handle
between the mouth and the belly. This ewer
shows strong Persian style of Sassanid Empire.
Preserved in Hebei Museum

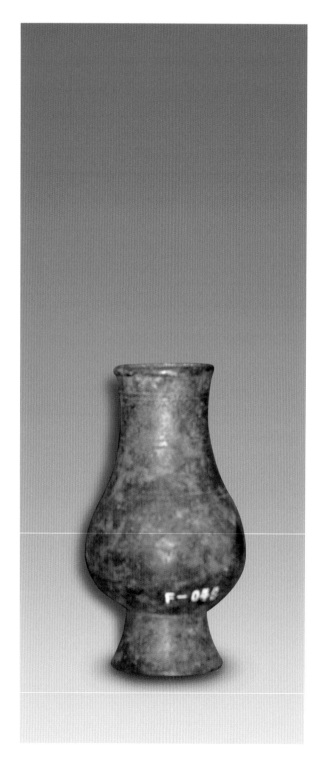

铜觯

唐

铜质

口径 5.4 厘米，底径 6.9 厘米，通高 15.5 厘米，重 500 克

Bronze Zhi Wine Vessel

Tang Dynasty

Bronze

Diameter 5.4 cm/ Bottom Diameter 6.9 cm/ Height 15.5 cm/ Weight 500 g

圆口，直颈，倒喇叭形座，周身线刻画绘。为
酒器。陕西省咸阳市征集。二十世纪七十年代
入藏。

陕西医史博物馆藏

The collection has a round mouth, a straight
neck, and a base whose shape is like an inverted
trumpet. There are decorative patterns on its
surface. The wine container Zhi was collected
in Xianyang City, Shaanxi Province, during the
1970s.

Preserved in Shaanxi Museum of Medical History

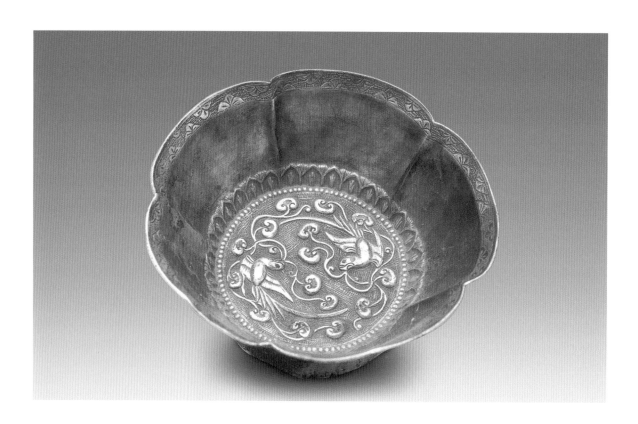

银碗

唐

银质

口径 11 厘米，底径 6.5 厘米，重 101 克

Silver Bowl

Tang Dynasty

Silver

Diameter 11 cm/ Bottom Diameter 6.5 cm/ Weight 101 g

平面花瓣形，侈口，折沿，平底。碗底阳刻

双鸟花卉图案，周边为一圈阴刻仰莲瓣纹。

武功县文物管理所藏

The petal-shaped bowl has a wide flared mouth, a folded rim, and a flat bottom. The bowl is engraved with birds and flowers at its bottom. Around the principal motifs at the bottom is a ring of lotus-petal designs.

Preserved in Wugong County Administration Office of Cultural Relics

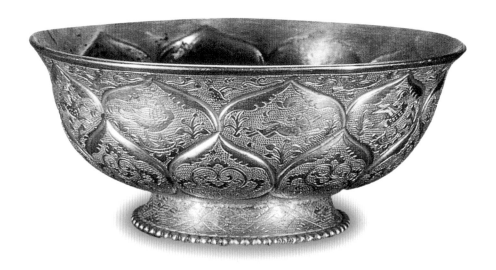

刻花赤金碗

唐

金质

口径 13.7 厘米，足径 6.7 厘米，高 5.5 厘米

Gold Bowl with Engraved Patterns

Tang Dynasty

Gold

Mouth Diameter 13.7 cm/ Bottom Diameter 6.7 cm/ Height 5.5 cm

口唇外撇，深腹弧壁，下接喇叭状的高圈足。碗外壁以上下两层错落分布的莲瓣为主题纹样，上层莲瓣之内，阴刻出折枝花卉及鸳鸯、鹦鹉、鹿、狐等珍禽异兽；下层莲瓣内刻有宝相花。莲纹之上是一周飞鸟流云，其下是一周锦簇团花。圈足外壁刻出菱形纹，足缘为一周连珠纹。所有纹饰均以鱼子纹为地。此碗线条流畅简约，装饰纹样丰富多彩，制作技法复杂精细，被视为稀世珍品。1970 年 10 月陕西省西安市何家村出土。

陕西历史博物馆藏

The bowl is widely open and deep with a ring base which looks like an inverted trumpet. Its exterior is decorated with two layers of lotus petals. There are Chinese ducks, parrots, deer and foxes in the upper layer petals while the low layer petals are filled with rosette designs. On the top of the two layers of lotus patterns, patterns of flying birds and clouds surround the exterior rim of the bowl. And the part underneath the petals is decorated with a cluster of flowers. The exterior wall of the ring foot is engraved with diamond patterns and a circle of pearl patterns surround the foot rim. All the motifs have fish patterns as their background. This bowl is regarded as a rare treasure in terms of its streamlined curve, various motifs, and complicated and delicate workmanship. It was unearthed at Hejiacun site, Xi'an City, Shaanxi Province, in October 1970.

Preserved in Shaanxi History Museum

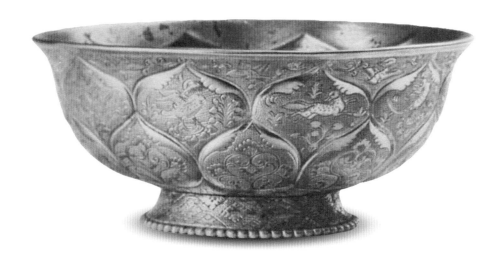

鎏金仰瓣荷叶圈足银碗

唐

鎏金银质

口径 16 厘米，足径 12.2 厘米，高 8 厘米，重 223 克

Gilt Silver Bowl with Lotus Petal Designs

Tang Dynasty

Gilt silver

Mouth Diameter 16 cm/ Foot Diameter 12.2 cm/ Height 8 cm/ Weight 223 g

钵呈扁圆形，唇口下沿部位饰二道细弦纹，鼓腹，平底。勺口呈椭圆形，扁柄细长弯曲自然。两件铜器虽然光素无纹，但铸造精良，器表光亮，造型给人一种稳重大方的感觉。钵、勺均为日常生活实用品。1964 年江苏省仪征市刘集村出土。

扬州博物馆藏

The bowl is oblate in shape with a bulged belly and a flat base. There are two rings of line patterns under its rim. The spoon is oval and its handle is long and curved. Although the bowl and the spoon are almost plain, they were well-made with shiny surface as well as poised and natural shape. Both of them were items for daily use. They were unearthed in Liuji County in Yizheng City, Jiangsu Province, in 1964. Preserved in Yangzhou Museum

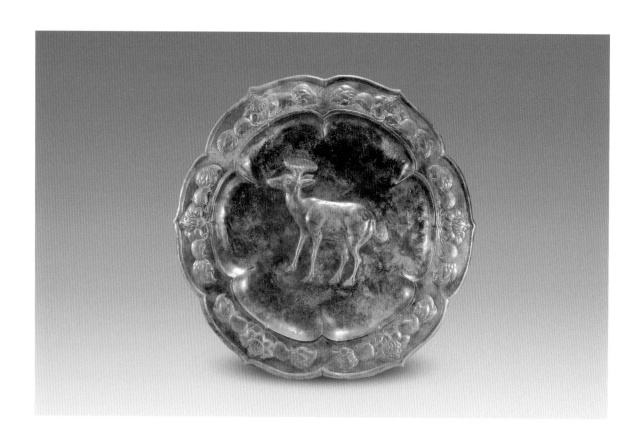

鎏金鹿纹菱花形银盘

唐

鎏金银质

口径 50 厘米，通高 10 厘米

Gilt Silver Linghua-shaped Plate with Deer Designs

Tang Dynasty

Gilt silver

Mouth Diameter 50 cm/ Height 10 cm

盘平面呈六瓣菱花形，敞口，宽折沿，浅腹，平底，卷叶状三足。盘心饰一凸起的梅花鹿。鹿头顶肉芝，身錾斑纹，四足前后错落。盘沿每瓣菱花内饰一组花卉。鹿和花卉表面鎏金。此盘器形硕大，做工精细，具有很强的立体感。

河北博物院藏

This plate, with a flared mouth, a shallow belly and a flat bottom, is in the shape of linghua flower with six petals. It has a wide folded rim and three leaf-shaped feet. In the center of the plate there is a convex deer engraved with patterns on its body and with a glossy ganoderma on the top of its head. The edge of the plate is decorated with flower clusters. The deer and flower groups are gilt. The plate is big and well-made.

Preserved in Hebei Museum

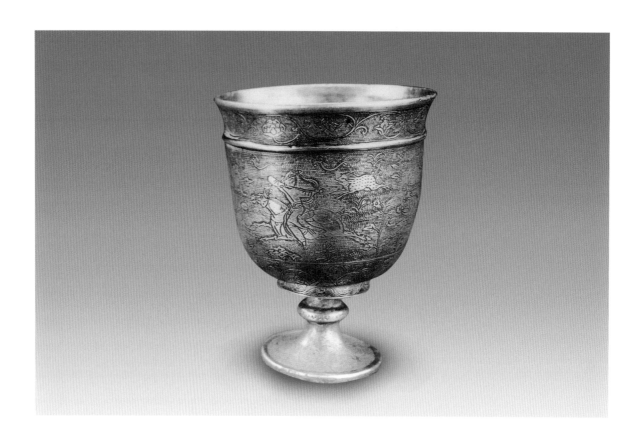

射猎纹高足银杯

唐

银质

口径 6 厘米，底径 3.4 厘米，高 7.3 厘米

Silver Goblet Patterned with Hunting Scene

Tang Dynasty

Silver

Mouth Diameter 6 cm/ Bottom Diameter 3.4 cm/ Height 7.3 cm

杯为侈口，深腹，高圈足。口沿、杯底及足
均饰缠枝花纹；腹部则饰有四幅射猎图，均
为射手骑在奔驰的马上，手握弓箭，追射惊
跑的野兽。1970年陕西省西安市何家村出土。

陕西历史博物馆藏

The deep goblet has a wide flared mouth and a
tall ring foot decorated with interlocking flower
patterns. On the exterior of the goblet are four
motifs which are scenes of hunting. The hunter
is riding on a galloping horse with a bow in
his hand chasing his game. The goblet was
unearthed at Hejiacun site, Xi'an City, Shaanxi
Province, in 1970.

Preserved in Shaanxi History Museum

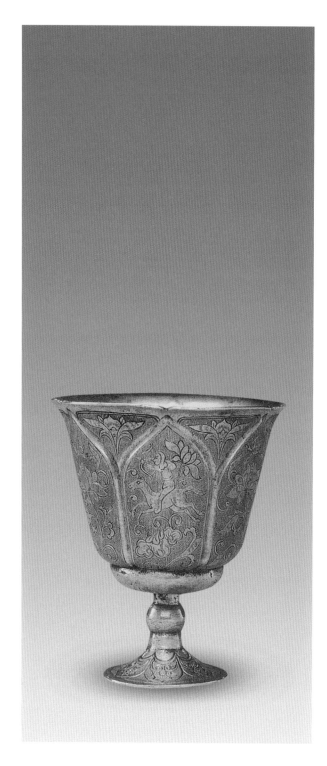

射猎莲瓣纹高足银杯

唐

银质

口径 6.9 厘米，高 7.8 厘米

Silver Goblet Patterned with Hunting Scene

Tang Dynasty

Silver

Mouth Diameter 6.9 cm/ Height 7.8 cm

杯为六曲侈口，斜直腹，高圈足。在腹部模
冲出的六枚尖莲瓣中，均有头戴风帽的骑士，
弯弓驰骋，呈射猎状。

美国弗利尔美术馆藏

The deep goblet has a wide flared mouth and a
tall ring foot. The cup is in the shape of a six-
petaled lotus. In each petal there is a hatted
hunter riding on a horse and hunting a game
with a bow.

Preserved in The Freer Gallery of Art, the United
States

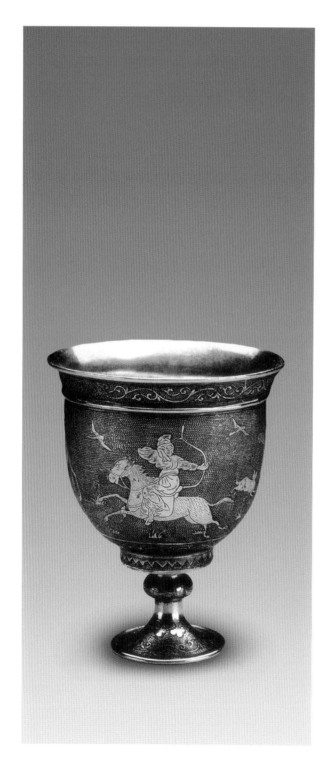

骑射纹银杯

唐

银质

通高 7.6 厘米

Silver Goblet Patterned with Riding and Shooting Scene

Tang Dynasty

Silver

Height 7.6 cm

侈口，口沿下一周突棱，深腹，高圈足。外壁口沿至突棱间饰缠枝花纹一周；腹部饰四幅骑射狩猎图，骑者均呈张弓欲射状，草丛中绘有惊恐逃奔的小兔。四幅骑射图的空间均填有花草和小鸟纹饰。

法国吉美国立亚洲艺术博物馆藏

The deep goblet has a wide flared mouth and a tall ring foot. There is a ring of raised line under its orifice. Interlocking flower patterns surround the exterior wall to the raised line. The four principal motifs on the belly are the scene of riding and shooting. The hunter is about to shoot at the harewhich is running for its life in the grass. The four motifs are decorated with patterns of flowers and birds.

Preserved in Musée National des Arts Asiatiques-Guimet, France

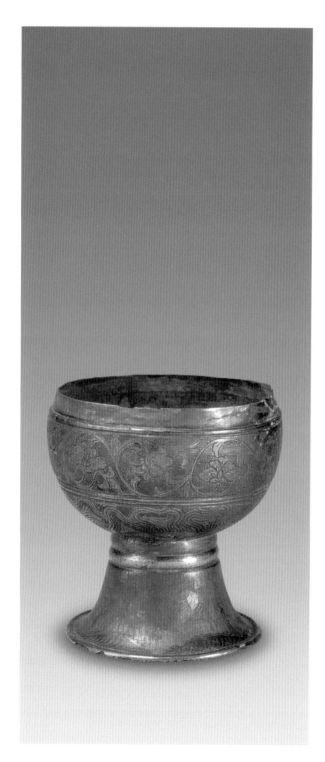

银高足杯

唐

银质

口径 8.5 厘米，底径 7.9 厘米，高 9.7 厘米

Silver Goblet

Tang Dynasty

Silver

Mouth Diameter 8.5 cm/ Bottom Diameter 7.9 cm/

Height 9.7 cm

敛口，口沿下一周突棱，鼓腹，高圈足。杯体的主题纹饰为缠枝牡丹与涡纹，圈足上的纹饰是荷叶纹上錾刻五只展翅的鸳鸯。刻工细腻，形态逼真，从形制看应属于晚唐时期。1980 年浙江省临安市唐水邱氏墓出土。

临安市文物馆藏

This goblet has a contracted mouth, a round belly, and a tall ring foot. There is a raised ring under its orifice. Its main motifs are interlocking peonies and scroll designs. Its base is engraved with lotus leaves and five fluttering Chinese ducks. The goblet boasts fine engraving work and lively form. Judging from its shape and structure, it should be a piece of work of the late Tang Dynasty. The goblet was unearthed from the tomb of Qiushi in Tangshui, Lin'an County, Zhejiang Province, in 1980.

Preserved in Lin'an Museum of Cultural Relics

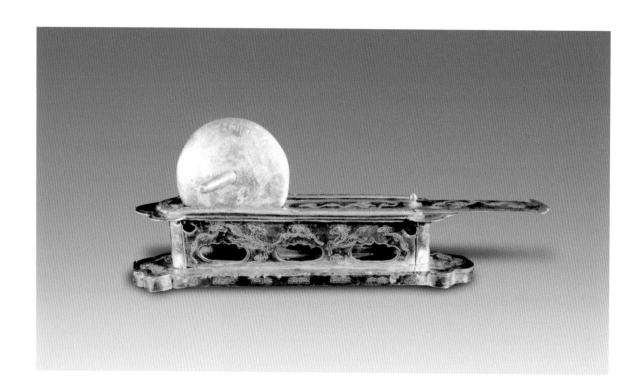

鎏金壶门座银茶碾子

唐

鎏金银质

碾槽：长 23.4 厘米，通高 7.1 厘米

碾轮：直径 8.9 厘米，轴长 21.6 厘米，重 1168 克

Gilt Silver Tea Roller with Arch-shaped Holes on the Base

Tang Dynasty

Gilt Silver

Base: Length 23.4 cm/ Height 7.1 cm

Roller: Wheel Diameter 8.9 cm/ Handle Length 21.6 cm/ Weight 1,168 g

通体长方形，由碾槽、辖板、槽座、碾轮四部分组成。碾槽呈半月尖底，连接于槽座，座有壶门，饰天马流云纹，座口有可抽动的辖板，不用时能够关闭。为碾制茶叶的专用器物。陕西省宝鸡市法门寺地宫出土。

法门寺博物馆藏

This rectangular artifact is composed of a roller and a base. The half-moon-shaped groove of the roller was welded onto the base decorated with arch-shaped holes accompanied by patterns of winged horses and clouds. The flexible bottom of the base can be closed when not in use. The roller was used exclusively for grinding tea. It was unearthed in the underground palace of Famen Temple, Baoji city, Shaanxi Province. Preserved in Famen Temple Museum

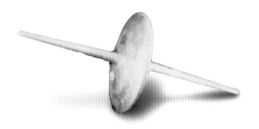

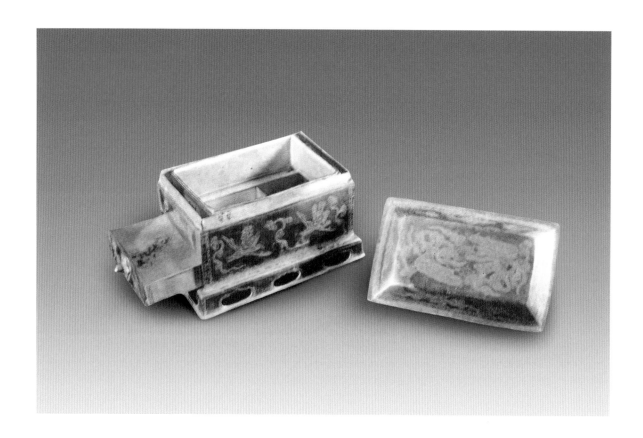

鎏金仙人驾鹤纹壶门座银茶罗子

唐

鎏金银质

长 13.4 厘米，宽 8.4 厘米，通高 9.5 厘米

Gilt Silver Tea Sifter Patterned with Immortal Beings and Cranes

Tang Dynasty

Gilt Silver

Length 13.4 cm/ Width 8.4 cm/ Height 9.5 cm

整体呈方形，由盖、罗、屉、罗架、器座五部分组成。罗架中上层为罗，罗分内外两层，中夹罗网。罗架下层为屉，以盛罗下之茶粉。罗架连接于壶门座上。华美精巧。陕西省宝鸡市法门寺地宫出土。

法门寺博物馆藏

This sifter is cuboid in shape. It consists of a lid, a sifter, a drawer, a frame, and a base. The frame, composed of two layers, was welded onto the base decorated with arch-shaped holes. The lower layer is the drawer as the container of the tea powder, and right on the top of it is the sifter. This delicate artifact was unearthed in the underground palace of Famen Temple in Baoji City, Shaanxi Province.

Preserved in Famen Temple Museum

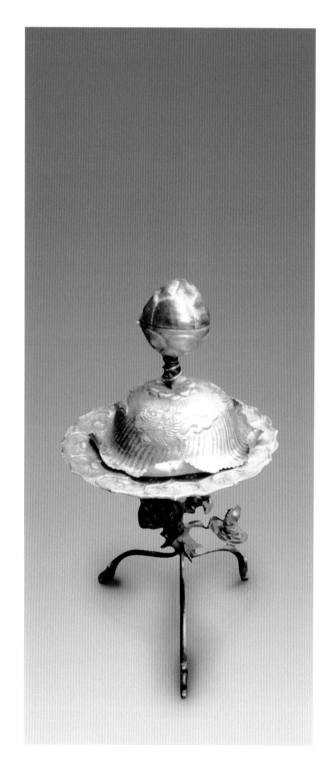

鎏金摩羯纹蕾钮三足银盐台

唐

鎏金银质

通高 25 厘米

Gilt Silver Salt Disk with Flower Designs and Tripod

Tang Dynasty

Gilt Silver

Height 25 cm

由盖、台盘、三足架组成。盖上有花蕾提手，中空，有铰链可以开合；下与盖连，盖沿如卷边荷叶。下为六盘，盘下连接三足支架。盘中用以盛盐，以调茶味。陕西省宝鸡市法门寺地宫出土。

法门寺博物馆藏

The salt disk is composed of a lid, a dish, and a tripod. The flower-bud-shaped lid knob itself is a container with its own lid connected with its lower part by a hinge. The edge of the lid curls upward, which makes the lid look like a lotus leaf. The dish was welded onto the tripod. Salt in the dish was the seasoning added to tea. This artifact was unearthed in the underground palace of Famen Temple in Baoji City, Shaanxi Province.

Preserved in Famen Temple Museum

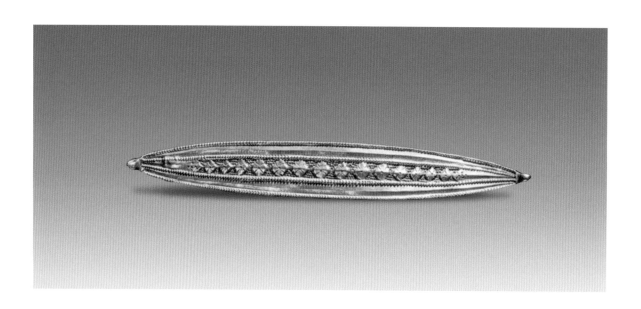

金发饰

唐

金质

长 15.9 厘米，宽 2 厘米，重 25.5 克

柳叶形，中间宽，两端渐收，端尖为一圆环。背面平整光素。正面纹饰錾刻而成，边缘饰连珠纹。中间饰以连珠纹为框，小圆点衬底，上饰一排菱形花朵组成的装饰图案。

山西博物院藏

Gold Hair Accessory

Tang Dynasty

Gold

Length 15.9 cm/ Width 2 cm/ Weight 25.5 g

The hair accessory, which is in the shape of a willow leaf, is wide in the middle and narrow at both ends. There is a ring at each end. The reverse side is smooth and plain, while the obverse side is highly decorated with carvings. The edges are carved with patterns of a string of pearls. The middle, between the two lines of strings of pearls, is filled with diamond-shaped flowers and small dots as background designs.

Preserved in Shanxi Museum

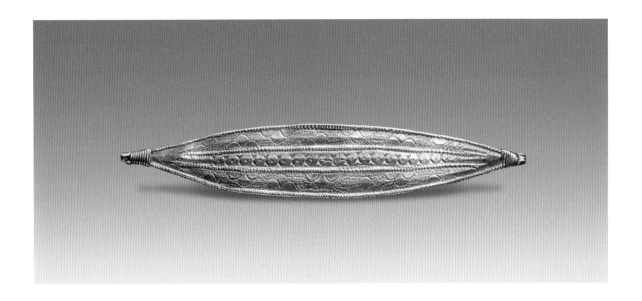

金发饰

唐

金质

长 14.7 厘米，宽 2.5 厘米。重 35.6 克

柳叶形，中间宽，两端渐收，端尖成丝，弯曲成
环后缠绕两端。背面平整光素。正面纹饰錾刻而
成，边饰连珠纹，中间饰以连珠纹为框，间饰同
心圆组成的图案，两边纹饰相同，为小圆点衬底，
扇形半圆组成几何图形。

山西博物院藏

Gold Hair Accessory

Tang Dynasty

Gold

Length 14.7 cm/ Width 2.5 cm/ Weight 35.6 g

The hair accessory, which is in the shape of a
willow leaf, is wide in the middle and narrow at
both ends. Each filamentous end curves to form a
ring before it intertwines toward the main body. The
reverse side is smooth and plain, while the obverse
side is highly decorated with carvings. The edges
are decorated with pearl designs. In the middle
there is a line of concentric circles, framed by two
strings of pearls. Other segments are patterned with
semicircles and dots as the background.

Preserved in Shanxi Museum

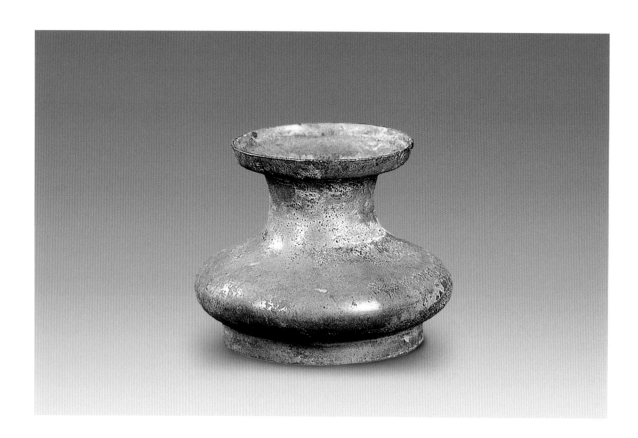

唾壶

唐

铜质

口径 6 厘米，底径 6.5 厘米，高 6.5 厘米

Spittoon

Tang Dynasty

Bronze

Mouth Diameter 6 cm/ Bottom Diameter 6.5 cm/ Height 6.5 cm

盘口，高颈，扁鼓腹，圜底，圈足。表面光亮，
略有锈蚀。河南省洛阳市出土。

上海中医药博物馆藏

The spittoon has a dish-shaped opening, a long
neck, a flat belly, a round bottom, and a ring
foot. Its surface is still shiny except for rusty
spots. The spittoon, a burial item, was unearthed
in Luoyang City, Henan Province.
Preserved in Shanghai Museum of Traditional
Chinese Medicine

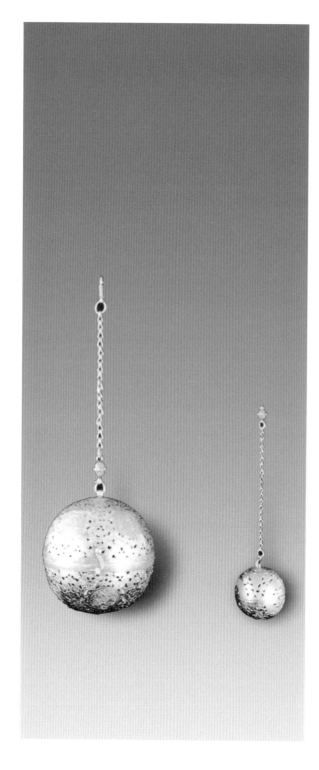

鎏金双锋团花纹镂孔银香囊（大）鎏金鸿雁纹镂孔银香囊（小）

唐

银质

大者：直径 12.8 厘米，链长 24.5 厘米，重 547 克

小者：直径 2.8 厘米，链长 17.7 厘米，重 87 克

Gilt Silver Incense Boxes

Tang Dynasty

Silver

The bigger one: Diameter 12.8 cm/ Length of the

Chain 24.5 cm/ Weight 547 g

The smaller one: Diameter 2.8 cm/ Length of the

Chain 17.7 cm/ Weight 87 g

两香囊均呈球体状，分上、下两半，可以开合。下半球内有两个同心圆组成的持平环，环中有香盂，可盛放香料。香囊结合后，可以任意滚动，而燃烧之香料不会倒出香盂。陕西省宝鸡市法门寺地宫出土。

法门寺博物馆藏

Both of the boxes, made in the shape of a ball, consist of two parts which can be opened. In the lower part, there are two rings supporting an incense container. The two rings keep the balance of the container so that incense will not spill out while the box is moving. The boxes were unearthed from the underground palace of Famen Temple in Baoji City, Shaanxi Province. Preserved in Famen Temple Museum

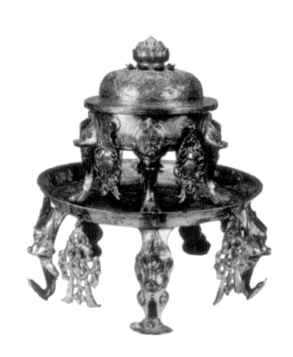

鎏金卧龟莲花纹五足银熏炉

唐

银质

盖径 25.9 厘米，腹深 7 厘米，通高 48 厘米，重 5363 克

Gilt Sliver Five-legged Incense Burner

Tang Dynasty

Silver

Lid Diameter 25.9 cm/ Belly Depth 7 cm/ Height 48 cm/ Weight 5,363 g

熏炉分炉盖、炉身和炉足三部分，炉盖面高隆，盖顶托一朵大莲蕾为盖钮，莲蕾下的覆莲座的各莲瓣向上半翘，形成一周熏炉的出烟孔。炉身碗状，腹外壁铆接五只炉足，足根为兽面，足为兽爪状。在足与足之间，又垂饰朵带，即打成花结的绶带。是唐代专为宫廷制造金银器的宫廷作坊文思院的产品，外形精美。1987 年陕西省宝鸡市法门寺地宫出土。

法门寺博物馆藏

The incense burner is composed of a lid, a container, and a base. The knob of the tall lid is in the shape of a big lotus bud on a lotus base with holes as outlet of the smoke. The container resembles a bowl with five legs in the shape of animal's legs. The upper part of each leg is decorated with animal designs and the lower part is in the shape of a claw. Pendent ribbons with flower knots are hung among the legs. This incense burner was made by the royal workshop, which produced gold and silver items for the imperial court in the Tang Dynasty. The extravagant and delicate artifact was excavated from the underground palace of Famen Temple in Baoji City, Shaanxi Province, in 1987.

Preserved in Famen Temple Museum

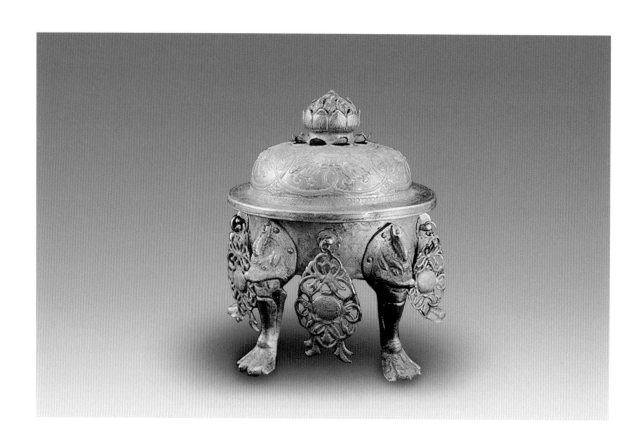

鎏金卧龟莲花纹朵带五足银熏炉

唐

银质

盖径 25.9 厘米，腹深 7 厘米，通高 29.5 厘米，重 5363 克

Gilt Sliver Five-legged Incense Burner

Tang Dynasty

Sliver

Lid Diameter 25.9 cm/ Belly Depth 7 cm/ Height 29.5 cm/ Weight 5,363 g

由炉盖、炉身两部分组成。炉盖面上有五朵莲花，各花花心卧有一只龟，中有莲瓣相托的宝珠盖钮，下层莲瓣镂空，以便香烟溢出。炉身周围有独角天龙足五个，两足间饰有朵带。外形精美。陕西省宝鸡市法门寺地宫出土。

法门寺博物馆藏

The whole burner is composed of a lid and a container. The lid is decorated with five lotuses with a turtle in the middle of each. The knob of the lid is a lotus bud sitting on a lotus base whose petals have holes as outlets of the smoke. The container sits on the feet of five unicorns. Among the feet, there are beautiful ribbons with exquisite flower knots as decoration. The incense burner was excavated from the underground palace of Famen Temple in Baoji City, Shaanxi Province.

Preserved in Famen Temple Museum

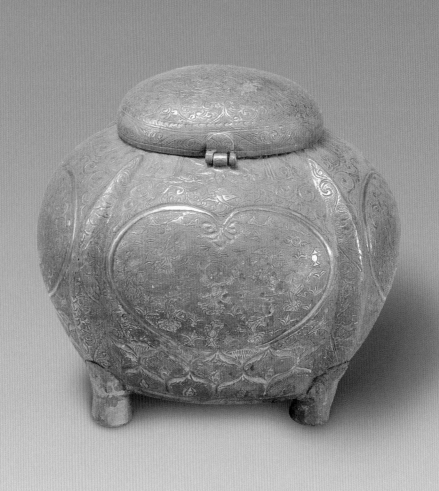

银盖罐

晚唐

银质

高 14.2 厘米

平面略方，四角圆转，平底下设四个对称的叶形圆柱足。盖沿与器肩两侧分别铆焊铰链、搭襻，可以落锁。通体鎏金。

临安市文物馆藏

Silver Jar with Lid

Late Tang Dynasty

Silver

Height 14.2 cm

This gilt jar is slightly cube-shaped. There are four leaf-shaped symmetrical feet under its bottom. The jar and its lid are linked by a hinge where a lock can be put in.

Preserved in Lin'an Museum of Cultural Relics

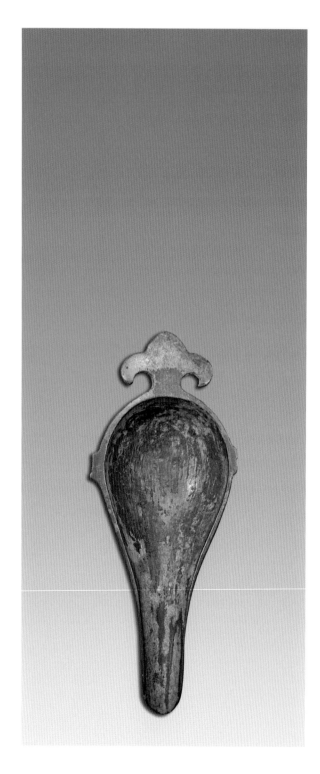

灌药器

唐末宋初

青铜

长 9 厘米，宽 9 厘米

Drencher

Late Tang and Early Song Dynasty

Bronze

Length 9 cm/ Width 9 cm

瓢形，云头纹执柄，弧形凹槽状长流，流端便于送药。做工精细，器型厚重，为中医早期急救器具。

张雅宗藏

The gourd ladle-shaped drencher was a medical device used in emergency in early time of Traditional Chinese Medicine. It has a handle with cloud patterns and a long arc groove, the end of which was used to deliver drugs. The drencher shows exquisite workmanship as well as thick and heavy material.

Collected by Zhang Yazong

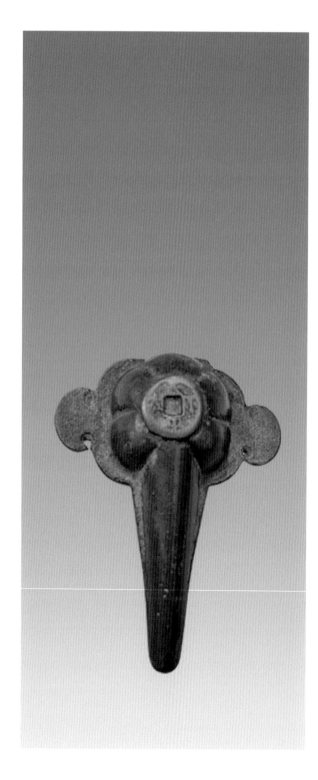

灌药器

唐末宋初

青铜

长 7.2 厘米，宽 5.6 厘米

Drencher

Late Tang and Early Song Dynasty

Bronze

Length 7.2 cm/ Width 5.6 cm

上端为池形盛药端，南瓜形腹，侈口，双耳，方孔币形底，刻有花纹。下端为扁平凹槽状长流，流端便于撬开牙齿输送药物。做工精细。为中医早期急救器具。

张雅宗藏

The drencher was a medical device used to rescue patients in emergency in early time of Traditional Chinese Medicine. It has a pumpkin-shaped belly, a wide flared mouth, two ears, a coin-shaped base with a square hole, and curved flower patterns. The pool-shaped upper end is used for holding the drug while the lower end is a flat and long groove for delivering the drug to an opened mouth. The drencher shows exquisite workmanship.

Collected by Zhang Yazong

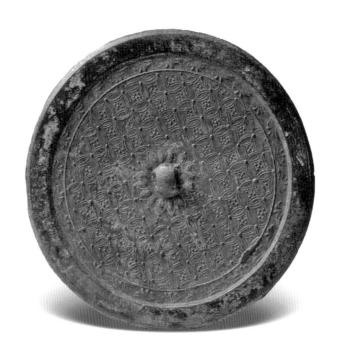

织锦连钱纹铜镜

五代

铜质

直径 18.2 厘米

Bronze Mirror with Brocade and Coin Designs

Five Dynasties

Bronze

Diameter 18.2 cm

圆形。鼻钮。钮外饰一周莲花瓣纹，外区
满饰细双线连方织锦钱纹，素缘。

南京市博物馆藏

The round mirror has a knob in the shape of
a bridge. The knob base is a circle of lotus
designs. The outer segment of the mirror is
decorated with double-line brocade coins
patterns while its edge is plain.

Preserved in Nanjing Municipal Museum

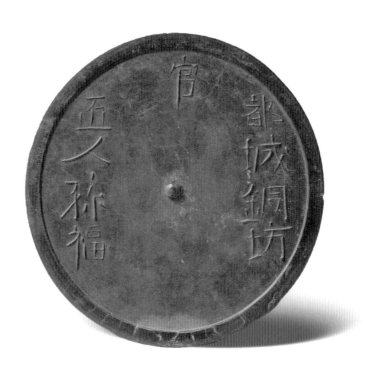

都城铜坊镜

五代

铜质

直径 18.8 厘米

Mirror marked with "Du Cheng Tong Fang"

Five Dynasties

Bronze

Diameter 18.8 cm

圆形。圆钮，花瓣纹钮座。纹饰分三圈，内圈为八卦纹，中圈为十二生肖，外圈为缠枝花。内圈有铭文置于八卦纹间，共八字，为"武德军作院罗真造"。"武德军作院"为前蜀武德军所设作坊。1983年四川巴中出土。

四川博物院藏

The round mirror has a hemispherical knob on the base with petal designs. The ornamentation includes three circular regions. The inner region is decorated with the design of the Eight Diagrams, the middle region is patterned with the Chinese zodiacs, and the outer region is filled with patterns of interlocking flowers. There are eight Chinese characters among the Eight Diagrams in the inner region, indicating the name of the workshop where it was made. The mirror was unearthed in Bazhong City, Sichuan Province, in 1983.

Preserved in Sichuan Museum

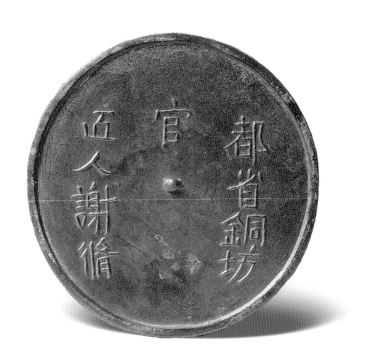

都省铜坊镜

五代

铜质

直径 18.4 厘米

Mirror marked with "Du Sheng Tong Fang"

Five Dynasties

Bronze

Diameter 18.4 cm

圆形。圆钮。镜背中央铸"官"字铭文，镜背顺列"都省铜坊"及"匠人谢修"款，字体率意，别具一格。传南京市南郊出土。

南京市博物馆藏

The round mirror has a hemispherical knob. The character above the knob means "official". The eight characters cast on its back in elegant and unique calligraphy are the names of the workshop and the workman. It is believed that the mirror was excavated on the southern suburbs of Nanjing City.

Preserved in Nanjing Municipal Museum

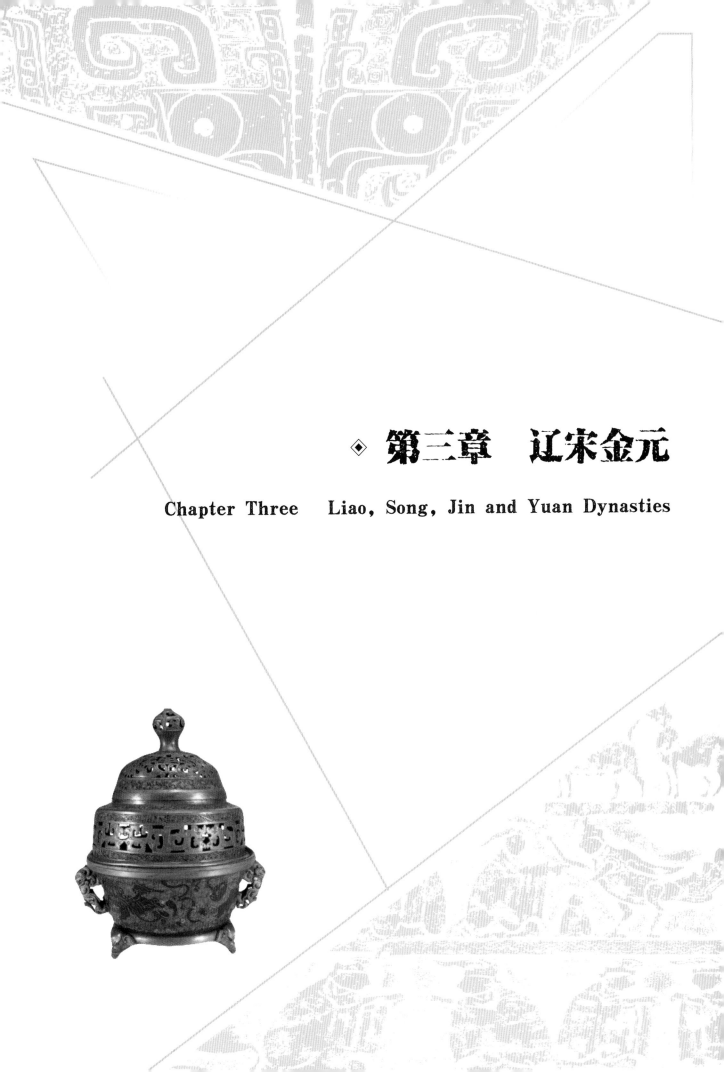

◇ 第三章 辽宋金元

Chapter Three Liao, Song, Jin and Yuan Dynasties

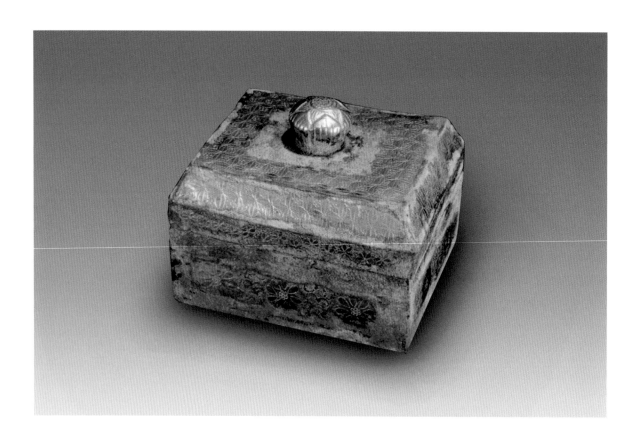

鎏金錾花刻经铜函

辽

铜质

长 17.2 厘米，宽 14.3 厘米，通高 13.5 厘米

Gilt Sutra Box

Liao Dynasty

Bronze

Length 17.2 cm/ Width 14.3 cm/ Height 13.5 cm

函呈长方形，盝顶形盖，通体鎏金。上有一
莲苞状钮，钮上錾单瓣仰莲纹，盖面饰钱纹，
花卉纹。函体四壁錾鱼子纹地，上饰莲花纹。
函内装《方广大壮严经》铜板 12 块，经板
为活页式，刻经文面鎏金。

河北博物院藏

This box is made in a cuboid shape. Both the
box and its terraced lid are gilt. The knob of
the lid resembles a lotus bud. The lid itself is
decorated with patterns of coins and flowers.
Lotuses are the principal motifs of the box with
small dots as the background. There are twelve
gilt bronze plates which are engraved with sutra
"Fang Guang Da Zhuang Yan Jing", a Buddhist
scripture.

Preserved in Hebei Museum

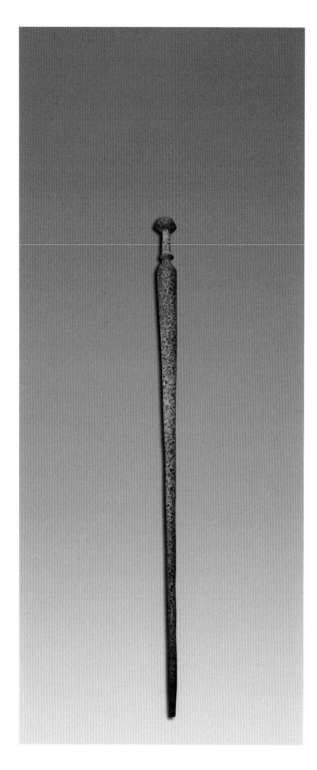

青铜针簪

辽

铜质

长 10.3 厘米，径 1.5 厘米

Bronze Needle

Liao Dynasty

Bronze

Length 10.3 cm/ Diameter 1.5 cm

相当于九针中的长针。细长针状，蘑菇形首。多见于辽代，后随针灸治疗技术的发展和演化逐渐减少。

张雅宗藏

The artifact, also known as the long needle among the 9 types of medical needles in Traditional Chinese Medicine, has a slender shape and a mushroom-like head. It was mainly seen in Liao Dynasty, but with the development of acupuncture technology it was used gradually less.

Collected by Zhang Yazong

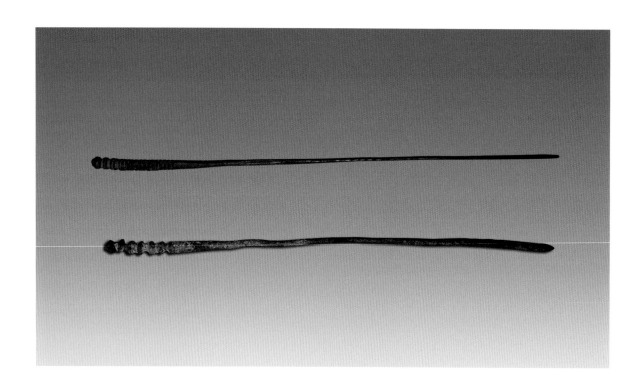

青铜针簪

辽

铜质

其一：长 14.5 厘米，径 1.5 厘米

其二：长 13.9 厘米，径 1.5 厘米

Bronze Needles

Liao Dynasty

Bronze

Needle One: Length 14.5 cm/ Diameter 1.5 cm

Needle Two: Length 13.9 cm/ Diameter 1.5 cm

两枚。相当于九针中的长针。细长针状，多节凸棱状柄。多见于辽代，后随针灸治疗技术的发展和演化逐渐减少。

张雅宗藏

The artifacts, also known as the long needle among the 9 types of medical needles in Traditional Chinese Medicine, have a slender shape and a mushroom-like handle with multiple protruded edges. It was mainly seen in Liao Dynasty, but with the development of acupuncture technology it was used gradually less.

Collected by Zhang Yazong

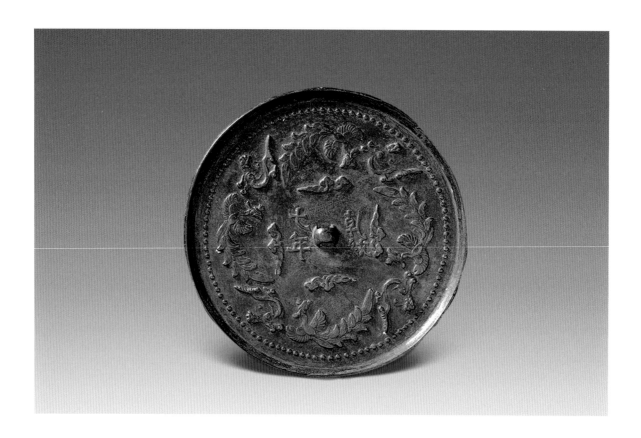

乾统七年镜

辽

铜质

直径 19 厘米

Mirror of the Seventh Year of Qiantong Period

Liao Dynasty

Bronze

Diameter 19 cm

圆形。圆钮。钮左右两侧铸"乾统七年"四字，钮上方刻"都右院官押"字样，外环饰四朵如意形祥云。主纹为长颈展翅飞翔的四凤纹，相间飞龙四条，外围连珠纹一周。乾统是辽天祚耶律延喜年号，乾统七年即公元1107年。

中国国家博物馆藏

The mirror is circular in shape with a hemispherical knob. Both sides of the knob are carved with characters indicating that the mirror was made in the seventh year of Qiantong Period (1107) in the Liao Dynasty. Its principal motifs consist of four auspicious clouds, four flying phoenixes and four dragons. The outside pattern is a ring of raised pearls.

Preserved in National Museum of China

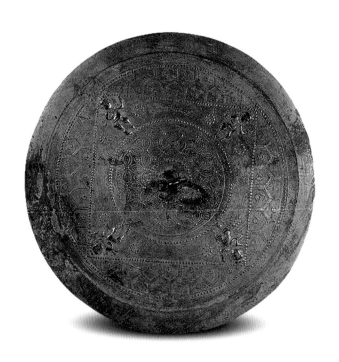

四童龟背纹镜

辽

铜质

直径 15 厘米

Mirror Patterned with Four Children and Turtlebacks

Liao Dynasty

Bronze

Diameter 15 cm

圆形。环钮，连珠纹钮座，座外饰四瓣花纹。
内区为方形，以连珠纹为界，四角各饰一童
子，神态各异；外区饰龟背纹。素宽边缘。
1957 年，辽宁省建平县张家营子出土。

辽宁省博物馆藏

The mirror is circular in shape and has a ring-shaped knob. The knob base is decorated with patterns of a chain of pearls and four-petaled flowers. A square divides the principal motifs into two regions. Four boys are standing in each corner of the square, and the outer region is filled with designs of turtlebacks. The edge is wide and plain. The mirror was unearthed at Zhangjiayingzi site in Jianping County, Liaoning Province, in 1957.

Preserved in Liaoning Provincial Museum

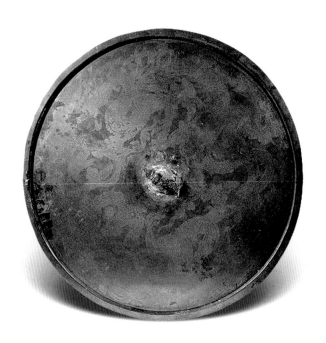

龙纹镜

辽

铜质

直径 38.5 厘米

Mirror with Dragon Designs

Liao Dynasty

Bronze

Diameter 38.5 cm

圆形。鼻钮。镜背用细线刻双龙绕钮飞舞，间饰卷云纹。此镜色泽亮洁，刻画精细，是辽镜中的佼佼者。1967 年，辽宁省阜新市塔子山辽塔地宫出土。

辽宁省博物馆藏

The mirror is circular in shape with a bridge-shaped knob. The principal motifs on the mirror's back are two dragons flying in clouds around the knob. The exquisite mirror is still shiny and is one of the best of all the mirrors unearthed in Liaoning Province. It was unearthed from the underground palace of a pagoda of Tazishan site in Fuxin City, Liaoning Province, in 1967.

Preserved in Liaoning Provincial Museum

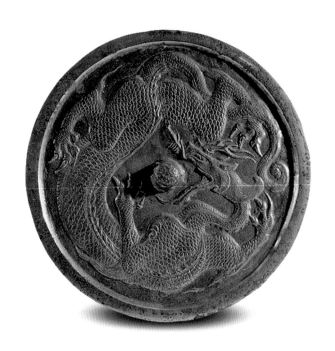

龙纹镜

辽

铜质

直径 28 厘米

Mirror with Dragon Designs

Liao Dynasty

Bronze

Diameter 28 cm

圆形。圆钮。镜背浮雕一盘龙，龙首昂起，双角耸立，张口吐舌，龙爪雄健有力，尾与一后足相纠结，通体饰鳞纹。1992 年内蒙古自治区赤峰市阿鲁科尔沁旗耶律羽之墓出土。

内蒙古自治区文物考古研究所藏

The mirror is circular in shape with a hemispherical knob. The principal motif on the back of the mirror is a coiled dragon in relief. The dragon is raising its head, holding its horns up, opening its mouth widely, and sticking out its tongue. Its claws are strong. Its tail entangles with one of its hind legs. Its body is covered with designs of scales. The mirror was unearthed from Yelü Yuzhi's tomb in Chifeng City, Inner Mongolia Autonomous Region, in 1992.

Preserved in Institute of Cultural Relics and Archaeology,Inner Mongolia

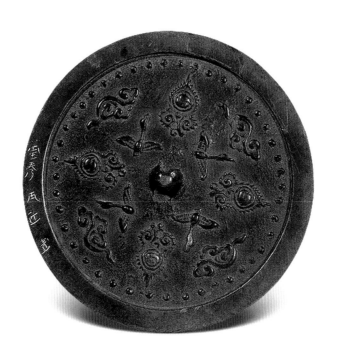

宝珠雁纹镜

辽

铜质

直径 12.3 厘米

Mirror Patterned with Precious Pearls and Wild Geese

Liao Dynasty

Bronze

Diameter 12.3 cm

圆形。圆钮。镜背主题纹饰为宝珠、大雁及云纹，雁均呈展翅飞翔状。近缘处饰乳钉纹一周，边缘上有金代刻女真文款及花押。

辽宁省博物馆藏

The mirror is circular in shape with a hemispherical knob. The principal motifs on the back are composed of pearls, flying wild geese and clouds, which are surrounded by a circle of nails. Nüzhen characters and marks are carved on the edge.

Preserved in Liaoning Provincial Museum

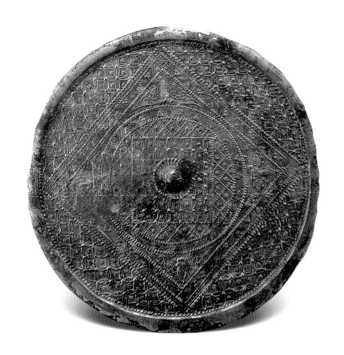

四蝶钱纹镜

辽

铜质

直径 29 厘米

Mirror Patterned with Butterflies and Coins

Liao Dynasty

Bronze

Diameter 29 cm

圆形。圆钮，连珠纹钮座。钮座外为连珠纹组成的方框，内饰连线纹。其外为连珠纹双圈与方框相交，圈内饰方块圈点纹。双圈又与连珠纹双线方框相切，方框四角饰四蝶展翅。其外饰连钱纹。1954 年内蒙古自治区赤峰市出土。

内蒙古博物院藏

The mirror is circular in shape with a hemispherical knob. The knob base is decorated with a chain of pearls. Outside of the knob base is a square filled with coin patterns. The square is enclosed by two circles of pearls, which are again encircled by three squares with a fluttering butterfly in each corner. Coin patterns were also used to decorate the exterior part of the bigger square. The mirror was unearthed in Chifeng City, Inner Mongolia Autonomous Region, in 1954.

Preserved in Inner Mongolia Museum

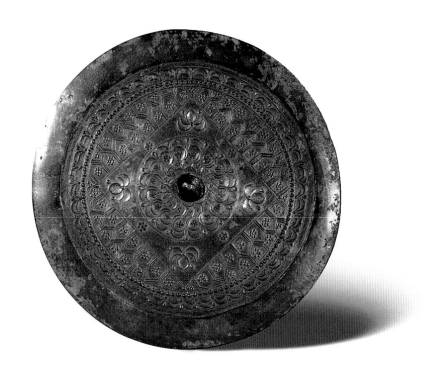

菊花龟背纹镜

辽

铜质

直径 19.5 厘米

Mirror Patterned with Chrysanthemum and Turtle Shells

Liao Dynasty

Bronze

Diameter 19.5 cm

圆形。圆钮，菊花纹圆钮座。内区呈方形，
四角各饰一花纹；外区饰龟背纹，其外饰连
珠纹重叠连弧纹各一周。此镜纹饰精细，是
辽镜中的精品。

辽宁省博物馆藏

The mirror is circular in shape with a hemispherical
knob. The knob base is decorated with
chrysanthemum designs. The principal motifs
are divided into two regions by a square with
a flower in each corner. The exterior region is
decorated with turtle shell designs, a ring of
pearls, and a ring of arc designs separately. The
mirror with exquisite patterns is the best of all
the mirrors unearthed in Liaoning Province.
Preserved in Liaoning Provincial Museum

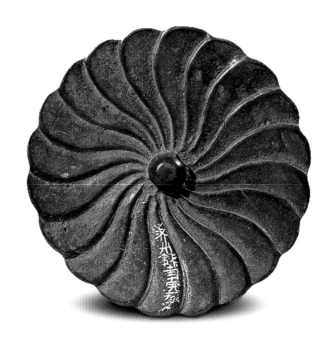

菊花纹镜

辽

铜质

直径 9.85 厘米

Mirror with Chrysanthemum Designs

Liao Dynasty

Bronze

Diameter 9.85 cm

菊花形。圆钮。镜背呈现菊花花瓣叠压旋转
的图案，极富动感。其中一花瓣上有金代刻
款"济州录司官"及花押。济州原名龙州，
金天眷三年（1140）改为济州，治所在利涉
县（今吉林省农安县）。

辽宁省博物馆藏

The mirror is circular in shape with a hemispherical
knob. Its back resembles chrysanthemum petals.
Five characters as inscriptions and the signature of
the official in charge of rituals in Jizhou are carved
on one flower petal. Jizhou, formerly known as
Longzhou, and it remaned to Jizhou in the 3nd
year of Tianjuan of Jin Dinasty (1140), used to be
the capital of Lishe State (now Nong'an county,
Jilin Province).

Preserved in Liaoning Provincial Museum

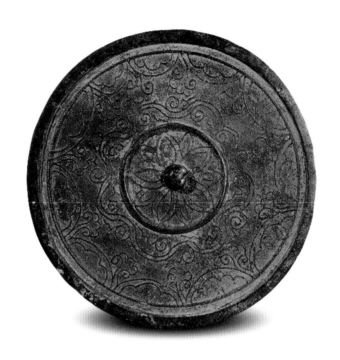

卷草花纹镜

辽

铜质

直径 17.6 厘米

Mirror with Flower Scroll Designs

Liao Dynasty

Bronze

Diameter 17.6 cm

圆形。圆钮，钮座内饰重瓣莲花。主题纹饰
为卷草花纹，双线勾画，委婉优雅，富流动感。
1967 年，辽宁省铁岭市有色金属熔炼厂出土。

辽宁省博物馆藏

The mirror is circular in shape with a hemispherical
knob. A raised ring divides its principal motifs
into two segments. The inner segment is
decorated with a double-petaled lotus, while the
outer segment is filled with flower scroll designs
in double lines. The mirror was unearthed from
a non-ferrous metal smelting plant of Tieling
City, Liaoning Province, in 1967.

Preserved in Liaoning Provincial Museum

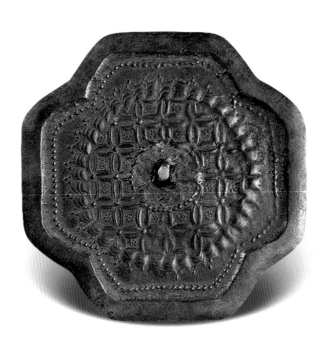

连钱锦纹"亞"形镜

辽

铜质

直径 10.9 厘米

Mirror with Coin Patterns

Liao Dynasty

Bronze

Diameter 10.9 cm

"亞"字形，桥形钮，连珠纹圆钮座。主题纹饰为连钱锦纹，每个钱孔内均有小花装饰。连钱外有三层叠压的花瓣装饰，边缘饰连珠纹一周。1967年，辽宁省铁岭有色金属熔炼厂出土。

辽宁省博物馆藏

The mirror is in the shape of a Chinese character "亞" and has a bridge-shaped knob. The knob base is round with a chain of pearls. Coin patterns are the principal motifs and are surrounded by a circle of arc patterns and a ring of pearls, with small flowers in each of the coin holes. The mirror was unearthed from a non-ferrous metal smelting plant of Tieling City, Liaoning Province, in 1967.

Preserved in Liaoning Provincial Museum

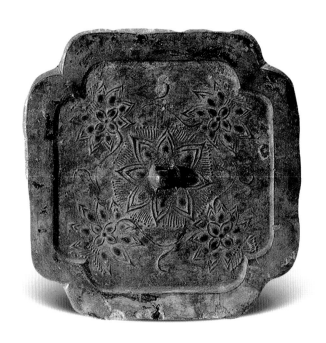

莲花纹"亚"形镜

辽

铜质

直径 15.8 厘米

Mirror with Lotus Patterns

Liao Dynasty

Bronze

Diameter 15.8 cm

"亞"字形。圆钮，花形钮座。四角各有一朵相同的莲花，花与花之间有枝相连。

湖南省博物馆藏

The mirror is in the shape of a Chinese character "亞" and has a hemispherical knob sitting on a base resembling a lotus. There is one lotus in each corner and all the lotuses are linked together by flower branches.

Preserved in Hunan Provincial Museum

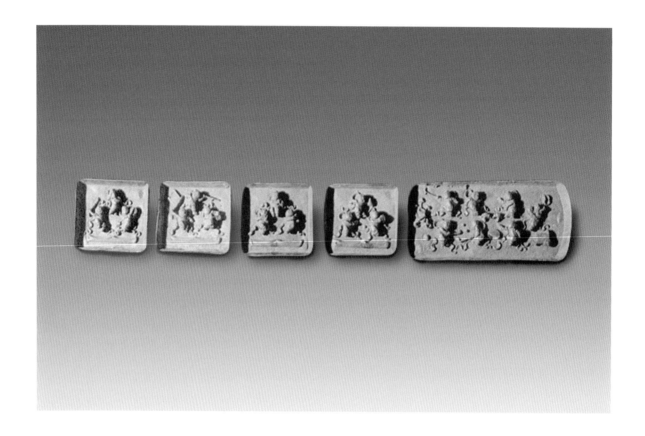

童戏纹鎏金银质大带

辽

银质

最大者长 13.6 厘米，宽 6.3 厘米

Silver Belts Patterned with Playing Children

Liao Dynasty

Maximum Length 13.6 cm/ Width 6.3 cm

大带共出土 5 块，其中小者 4 块，为正方形；大者 1 块为长方形。四周皆有折缘边框，框内采用焊接、铸印、锤揲等工艺各装饰了一组包括童子捶丸、弄风车以及舞蹈在内的游戏图案。1972 年辽宁省朝阳县前窗户村辽墓出土。

朝阳市博物馆藏

The belt consists of four small square pieces and one big rectangular piece. Each piece has a square rim in which a game design is decorated through welding, casting or hammering skills. The designs vary from piece to piece, mainly about kids playing with balls or pinwheels or dancing. The belt was excavated from a tomb of the Liao Dynasty in Chaoyang County, Liaoning Province, in 1972.

Preserved in Chaoyang Museum

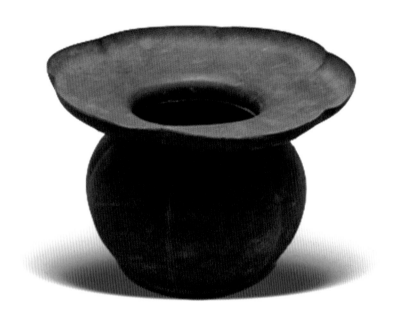

唾盂

辽

铜质

口径 29 厘米，高 15 厘米

Spittoon

Liao Dynasty

Bronze

Mouth Diameter 29 cm/ Height 15 cm

盘口，鼓腹，平底，盘沿为荷瓣纹，腹呈瓜
棱形。由民间征集。

成都中医药大学中医药传统文化博物馆藏

The spittoon has a dish-shaped mouth, a bulged
belly, and a flat bottom. The rim of the mouth
is decorated with designs of lotus leaves while
its belly resembles a melon. The spittoon was
collected from a private owner.

Preserved in Museum of Traditional Chinese
Medicine Culture, Chengdu University of
Traditional Chinese Medicine

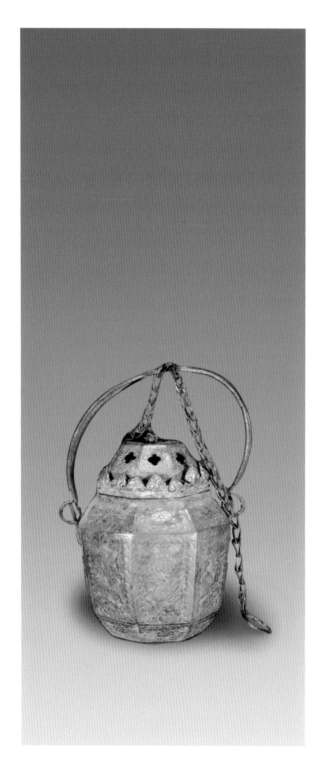

鎏金花鸟纹铜熏炉

辽

铜质

腹径 11.6 厘米，通高 14 厘米

Gilt Sliver Incense Burner Patterned with Flowers and Birds

Liao Dynasty

Bronze

Belly Diameter 11.6 cm/ Height 14 cm

敛口，圆唇，折肩，平底。通体鎏金。肩两侧各有一环，与弧形提梁相连接，梁顶中部有一长链，与盖面的环钮相连。盖呈八角僧帽状，上有镂孔，沿四周模压云形灵芝纹，肩及近底部各饰花卉纹一周，腹部錾刻精细的花鸟纹。

河北博物院藏

The whole burner is like an octagonal jar with a contracted mouth and a folded shoulder. A pair of loops connects with its arc-shaped handle. In the middle of the handle there is a long chain which links the ring knob of the octagonal lid. Holes on the lid are surrounded by patterns of clouds. The shoulder and the lower belly of the burner are decorated with flowers. The belly of the burner is decorated with patterns of flowers and birds.

Preserved in Hebei Museum

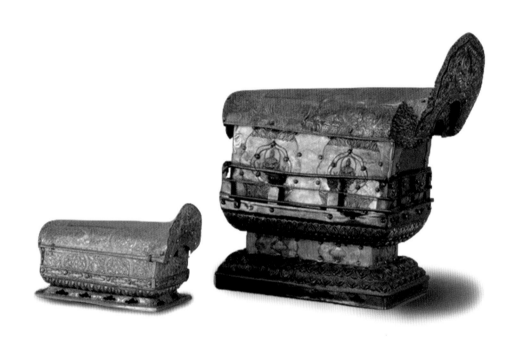

金棺银椁

北宋

金质

金棺：长 17.8 厘米，高 7.5~10.6 厘米，重 331.5 克

银椁：长 27.2 厘米，高 20.3~28.3 厘米，重 1005 克

金棺置于银椁内，二者的形制基本相同，均为长方匣形，带盖。表面均满饰花纹，金棺表面为花卉，银椁椁盖为花卉，椁身为包金的佛像。整个棺具玲珑别致，工艺绝伦。为盛装舍利子的专用器具。

武功县文物管理所藏

Gold Coffin with Silver Outer Coffin

Northern Song Dynasty

Gold and silver

Gold coffin: Length 17.8 cm/ Height 7.5-10.6 cm/ Weight 331.5 g

Silver outer coffin: Length 27.2 cm/ Height 20.3-28.3 cm/ Weight 1,005 g

The two exquisite and unique coffins are similar in shape. Both are oblong boxes with a cover and decorative designs. The gold one is placed inside the silver one. The gold coffin and the cover of the silver outer coffin are decorated with flowers, while the body of the silver outer coffin is patterned with Buddha overlaid with gold. They were dedicated containers for Buddha's relics.

Preserved in Wugong County Administration Office of Cultural Relics

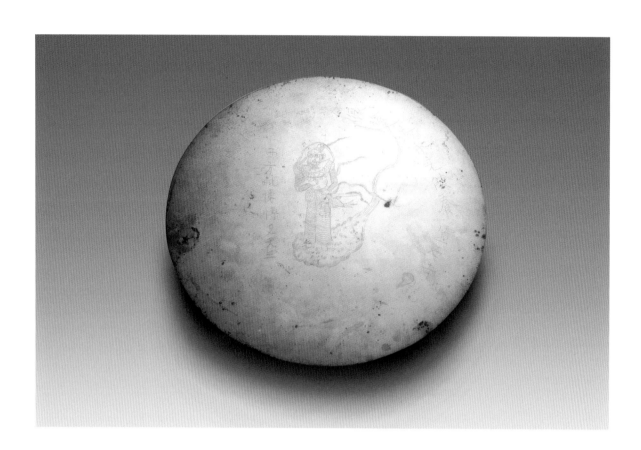

铜镜

北宋

铜质

直径 24.5 厘米

Bronze Mirror

Northern Song Dynasty

Bronze

Diameter 24.5 cm

椭圆形。镜背花鸟祥云，镜面细刻"西方毗楼博叉天王"像，镜周刻"乾德四年丙寅九月十五日勾当僧归进慕缘舍入塔永充供养灵石寺记"。

黄岩博物馆藏

The mirror is oval-shaped. Its back is decorated with flowers, birds and auspicious clouds. The portrait of Virupaksa, a god guarding the west, is carved on the surface of the mirror. Twenty-nine Chinese characters are also carved in a circle on the mirror, describing the time and the monk who enshrined the mirror.

Preserved in Huangyan Museum

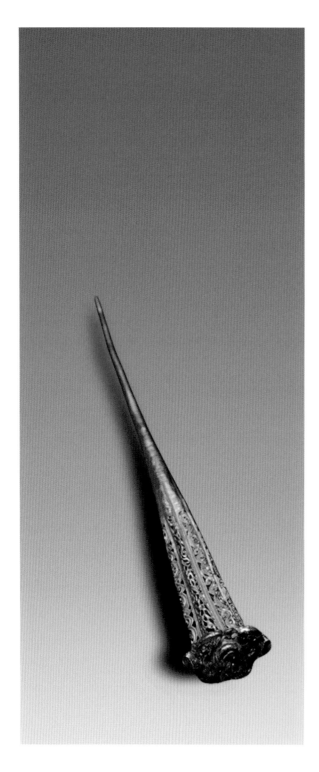

团龙金簪

北宋

金质

长 16.4 厘米

Gold Hairpin with Twining Dragon Patterns

Northern Song Dynasty

Gold

Length 16.4 cm

簪体呈圆锥形，簪顶中间錾刻一团龙，盘曲蜿蜒，四周等距离刻 6 枚灵芝，绕成圆形。簪体上部镂空雕 6 条长卷草纹。采用了錾刻、镂雕、焊接等工艺手法。南京市幕府山出土。

南京市博物馆藏

This hairpin is conical in shape. The top of the hairpin is carved into a twining dragon surrounded by six glossy ganodermas. The body of the hairpin consists of six long scroll design. Carving, hollow engraving and welding skills were used in making the hairpin. It was unearthed from Mount Mufu in Nanjing. Preserved in Nanjing Municipal Museum

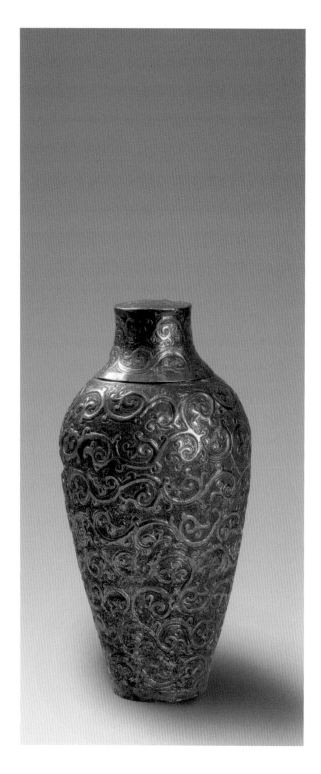

香草纹银瓶

南宋

银质

口径 4.2 厘米，底径 5.5 厘米，高 21.5 厘米

Silver Bottle

Southern Song Dynasty

Silver

Diameter 4.2 cm/ Bottom Diameter 5.5 cm/ Height

21.5 cm

盘口，短颈，丰肩，肩以下渐收腹至底，圈足。有盖，盖平顶呈喇叭状。瓶身及盖均饰蔓状香草纹，并錾以珍珠地纹。肩部錾刻凹香草纹一周和弦纹一道，盘口外刻一圈云雷纹。盖顶以四叶柿蒂纹为中心，周围配以缠枝草纹。瓶体修长，比例均匀，采用錾刻、焊接等工艺制作。南京江浦黄悦岭张同之墓出土。

南京市博物馆藏

The bottle has a dish-shaped mouth, a very short neck, a broad tapered shoulder, and a ring foot. Its lid resembles an inverted trumpet. Both the bottle and its lid are decorated with patterns of twining vines and small pearl designs as the background. A ring patterns surround the bottle's shoulder, while its dish-shaped opening is patterned with a ring of cloud and thunder designs. The top of the lid is covered with the persimmon pedicle patterns surrounded by twining vines. The slender and proportional bottle was made with techniques of carving and welding. The bottle was unearthed from the tomb of Zhang Tongzhi, in Nanjing.

Preserved in Nanjing Municipal Museum

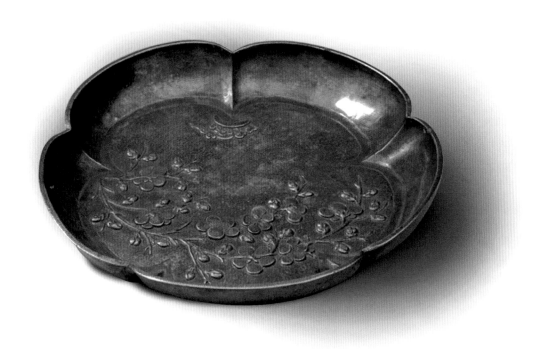

月影梅银盘

南宋

银质

直径 14.6 厘米，高 1.9 厘米

Silver Plate with Moon and Plum Designs

Southern Song Dynasty

Silver

Diameter 14.6 cm/ Height 1.9 cm

盘呈五瓣梅花形，平底。盘心錾刻一枝盛开的梅花及朵云托月纹饰，月光初照，疏影横斜，一派"暗香浮动月黄昏"的情境，极富诗意，构思独特别致。南京江浦黄悦岭张同之墓出土。

南京市博物馆藏

The plate is made in the shape of a five-petaled plum blossom, with a branch of plum tree and the moon in the mist of clouds on its flat bottom. The rising moon, the big dim shadows casted by the moon, and the hidden smell of fragrance all clearly and poetically describe that the dusk is gathering. The design of the plate is very unique and poetic. The plate was unearthed from the tomb of Zhang Tongzhi, in Nanjing.
Preserved in Nanjing Municipal Museum

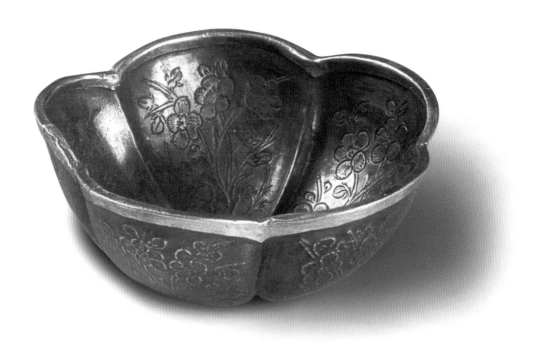

梅花形银盂

南宋

银质

口径 9.5 厘米，高 3.9 厘米

Silver Bowl with Plum Blossom Designs

Southern Song Dynasty

Silver

Mouth Diameter 9.5 cm/ Height 3.9 cm

盂呈五瓣梅花形，口沿包金皮，从口至底逐步收敛，圜底。整个造型犹似梅花盛开。盂心錾刻一朵凸出的梅花，且盂壁上分别錾刻有五枝折枝梅花。器物构思独特别致，纹饰华丽繁密，其装饰与造型达到了和谐统一。南京江浦黄悦岭张同之墓出土。

南京市博物馆藏

The bowl resembles a plum blossom with five petals. The mouth is widely open and its base is round and small. Its rim is covered with gold. A raised plum blossom is carved on the bottom. There is a branch of plum tree with flowers on each petal part of the bowl. This masterpiece of art is really magnificent with unique design and ornamentation. The bowl was unearthed from the tomb of Zhang Tongzhi, an official in the Northern Song Dynasty, in Nanjing.
Preserved in Nanjing Municipal Museum

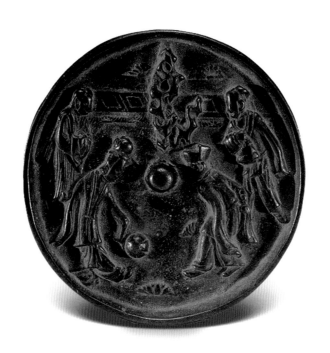

蹴鞠纹镜

南宋

铜质

直径 10.8 厘米

Mirror with Scene of Cuju Ball Playing

Southern Song Dynasty

Bronze

Diameter 10.8 cm

圆形。圆钮。主题纹饰为蹴鞠娱乐图，图中
一男一女正专心踢球，两侧饰男女二人及太
湖石、围墙、山峦等，其间饰以花草纹。湖
南省株洲市征集。

湖南省博物馆藏

The mirror is round in shape and its knob is
hemispherical. Its principal motif is a scene
of a man and a woman playing cuju ball, with
another man and another lady watching them.
The rest part of the scene is decorated with
ornamentations such as an artificial hill, a fence
and a mountain, among which are patterns of
flowers and grass. The mirror was collected in
Zhuzhou City, Hunan Province.
Preserved in Hunan Provincial Museum

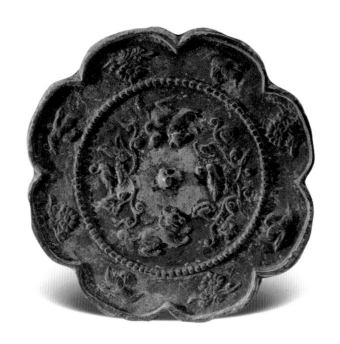

鸟兽纹葵花镜

南宋

铜质

直径 17.1 厘米

Mallow-shaped Mirror with Patterns of Animals and Birds

Southern Song Dynasty

Bronze

Diameter 17.1 cm

八瓣葵花形。圆钮。一圈凸起的连珠纹把镜
背分成两区，内区为对称的两兽和莲花小鸟；
外区为莲花与飞鸟相间排列。湖南省长沙市
征集。

湖南省博物馆藏

The mirror is in the shape of a mallow flower
with eight petals. Its knob is hemispherical. The
main motifs are divided into two segments by a
raised ring of pearls. The inner segment consists
of symmetric animals, lotuses and birds, while
the outer segment is decorated with four lotuses
and four birds. The mirror was collected in
Changsha City, Hunan Province.
Preserved in Hunan Provincial Museum

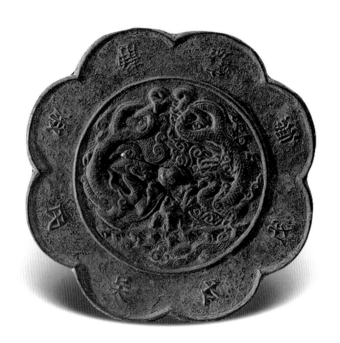

嘉熙戊戌双龙纹葵花镜

南宋

铜质

直径 19.5 厘米

Mallow-shaped Mirror with Double Dragons

Southern Song Dynasty

Bronze

Diameter 19.5 cm

八瓣葵花形。圆钮。一周凸弦纹把镜背分成两区，内区为双龙，下半部似岸边立一个三足香炉形器；外区为"嘉熙戊戌吴氏淑静"八字铭文，嘉熙戊戌为公元1238年。

湖南省博物馆藏

The mirror is in the shape of a mallow flower with eight petals. Its knob is hemispherical. A raised ring divides its principal motifs into two segments. Two dragons are in the inner segment with a three-legged incense burner between them. The outer segment is inscribed with eight characters as epigraph indicating the year (1238) when the mirror was made and its owner.
Preserved in Hunan Provincial Museum

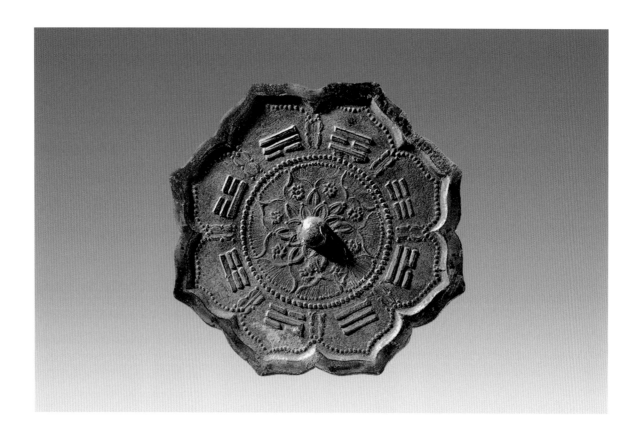

八卦菱花镜

南宋

铜质

直径 10.7 厘米

Linghua Flower Mirror with Patterns of the Eight Diagrams

Southern Song Dynasty

Bronze

Diameter 10.7 cm

八瓣菱花形。圆钮，菱花形钮座。主题纹饰为八瓣菱花内各饰一八卦符号。河南省洛阳市铁路一小出土。

洛阳博物馆藏

The mirror is in the shape of a linghua flower with eight petals. Its hemispherical knob sits on a base decorated with linghua flower designs. The Eight Diagrams is the principal motif on the back of the mirror. The mirror was unearthed in Luoyang City, Henan Province.

Preserved in Luoyang Museum

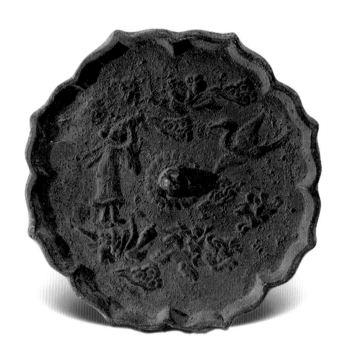

人物花鸟菱花镜

南宋

铜质

直径 12.8 厘米

Linghua Flower Mirror Patterned with Figures, Birds and Flowers

Southern Song Dynasty

Bronze

Diameter 12.8 cm

八瓣菱花形。圆钮，花形钮座。左边有一身
着长袍，一手伸到头部，站于玄武之上的人
仰首而望，上部为骑鹤之人飞翔于云层之中，
右边为展翅飞翔的仙鹤，下部有骑马奔跑的
人。湖南省株洲市征集。

湖南省博物馆藏

The mirror is in the shape of a linghua flower
with eight petals. Its hemispherical knob sits
on a flower-shaped knob base. On the left side
of the knob, a person in a robe standing on a
turtle is looking up at the sky with one of his
hands raised as high as his head. And in the sky
another person is flying on a crane in the clouds.
On the right side a crane is flying with its wings
fully spread. Below the knob a person is riding
a galloping horse. The mirror was collected in
Zhuzhou City, Hunan Province.
Preserved in Hunan Provincial Museum

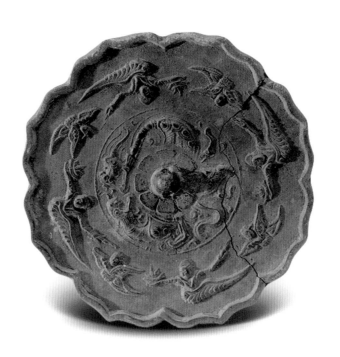

飞仙龙虎纹菱花镜

南宋

铜质

直径 11 厘米

Linghua Flower Mirror with Immortal, Dragon and Tiger Patterns

Southern Song Dynasty

Bronze

Diameter 11 cm

八瓣菱花形。圆钮，花形钮座。一周细小的
凸弦纹把镜背分成两区，内区为龙虎纹，外
区为飞翔的仙人。

湖南省博物馆藏

The mirror is in the shape of a linghua flower
with eight petals. Its hemispherical knob sits on
a flower-shaped knob base. A raised ring divides
the main motifs into two segments. The inner
segment is decorated with tiger and dragon
patterns while the outer segment is decorated
with flying immortals.

Preserved in Hunan Provincial Museum

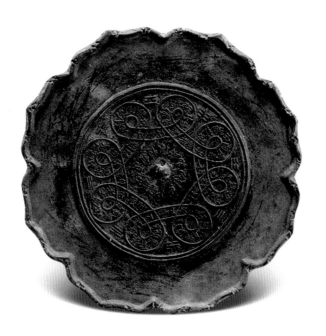

《满江红》词菱花镜

南宋

铜质

直径 21.7 厘米

Linghua Flower Mirror Cast with a Chinese Song Poem

Southern Song Dynasty

Bronze

Diameter 21.7 cm

八瓣菱花形。圆钮。由凸起的双弦纹组成一
圆圈，圈内两条平行线组成有八个回环的环
带，环带及钮周围录《满江红》词，从"雪
共梅花"起始到"须相忆"结束，共九十三字。
回环间置八卦纹。菱边有一圈梅花形凹槽，
当用于镶嵌。

北京市文物研究所藏

The mirror is in the shape of a linghua flower
with eight petals. It has a hemispherical knob.
Two raised rings separate the principal motifs
into two segments. In the inner region two
raised strings compose around the knob a ribbon
with eight loops. Man Jiang Hong (*Floating
Fern*), a Chinese song poem with 93 characters,
is cast on the ribbon and around the knob. The
inner region is decorated with patterns of the
Eight Diagrams. The edge of the mirror has a
round plum-shaped groove for inlaying.
Preserved in Beijing Municipal Institute of
Cultural Relics

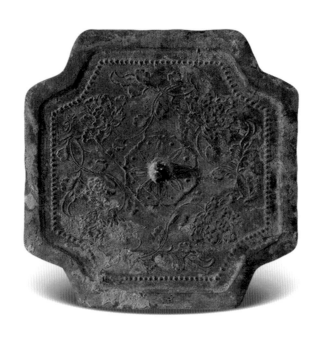

缠枝花"亞"形镜

南宋

铜质

直径 13.8 厘米

Mirror Patterned with Interlocking Flowers

Southern Song Dynasty

Bronze

Diameter 13.8 cm

"亞"字形。圆钮，花形钮座。钮座周围布
满缠枝花，外围"亞"字形的连珠纹。

湖南省博物馆藏

The mirror is in the shape of the Chinese
character "亞". It has a hemispherical knob and
the flower-shaped knob base is surrounded by
interlocking flowers. The edge of the mirror is
decorated with pearl patterns.

Preserved in Hunan Provincial Museum

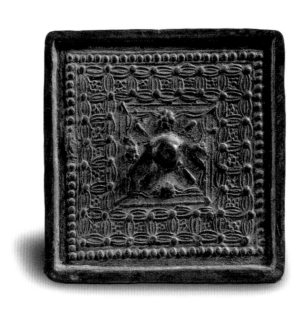

钱纹方镜

南宋

铜质

边长 8.3 厘米

Square Mirror with Coin Patterns

Southern Song Dynasty

Bronze

Side Length 8.3 cm

方形。圆钮。钮周围饰珠纹组成的花朵及四出纹，其外围以双线方框。主纹为连钱纹，钱孔内各置小花一朵，四角饰圆珠，圆珠相连成两个方框。四边由连珠纹组成。1957 年吉林省梨树县出土。

吉林省博物院藏

The mirror is square in shape. It has a hemispherical knob surrounded by four flowers in a double-lined square. The mirror is mainly decorated with coin patterns and in each coin hole there is a flower. There is a ball in each of the four corners of a coin and all the balls form two squares. The four sides of the mirror are decorated with a chain of pearls. The mirror was unearthed in Lishu County, Jilin Province, in 1957.

Preserved in Jilin Provincial Museum

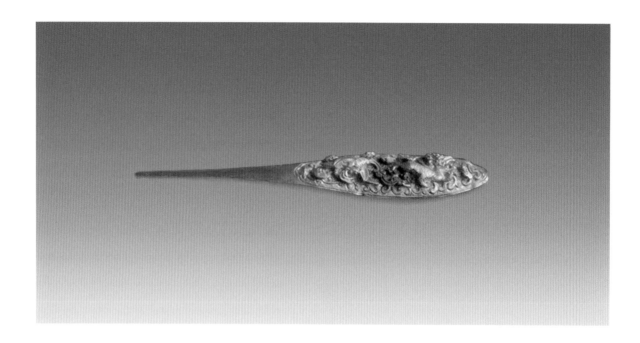

龙凤纹金簪

南宋

金质

长 17.4 厘米，宽 2.3 厘米

Gold Hairpin with Dragon and Phoenix Designs

Southern Song Dynasty

Gold

Length 17.4 cm/ Width 2.3 cm

扁平状，在簪体上半部锤压出龙、凤、灵芝、
如意云纹，再錾刻各纹饰的细部，做工考究。
在灵芝地纹上，飘缀如意祥云，飞龙眷顾，
舞凤相随，遨游嬉戏于云涛之间，寓意吉祥，
极富动感。显示了宋代金银工艺的高超技术。
南京幕府山出土。

南京市博物馆藏

The hairpin is flat. One end of it is decorated
with patterns of dragon, phoenix, glossy
ganoderma and auspicious floating clouds.
The dragon is flying happily, followed by an
elegant phoenix. The design implies something
propitious. This hairpin presents the first-rate
techniques of gold and silver ware making in
the Song Dynasty. The hairpin was unearthed
from Mount Mufu in Nanjing.
Preserved in Nanjing Municipal Museum

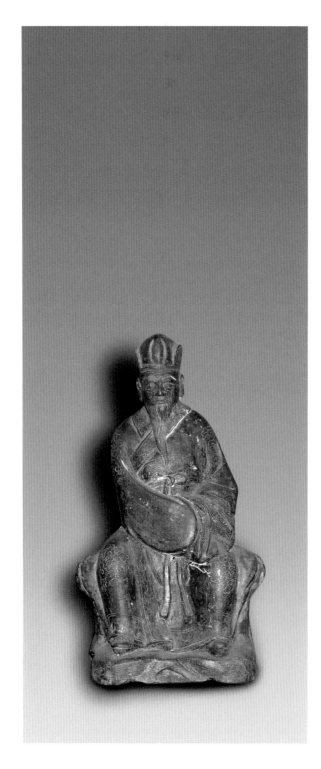

铜药王像

宋

铜质

底径 12.5 厘米，通高 25 厘米，重 1550 克

为一药王坐相的造像，头带官帽，身穿长袍，底
座有残。

陕西医史博物馆藏

Statue of the King of Medicine

Song Dynasty

Bronze

Bottom Diameter 12.5 cm/ Height 25 cm/ Weight
1,550 g

This statue is the King of Medicine in sitting
posture. He is wearing an official's hat and a robe.
The base is incomplete.

Preserved in Shaanxi Museum of Medical History

八卦星月纹串铃

宋

铜质

外径 12.5 厘米，内径 4 厘米

圆环形，表面满刻云纹，正面有日、月、叁星、北斗星像，反面为八卦卦像。内置铜丸四颗，摇动能发出铃声，是民间医生行医器具。

上海中医药博物馆藏

Bell Patterned with the Eight Diagrams

Song Dynasty

Bronze

Outer diameter 12.5 cm/ Inner diameter 4 cm

This bell is in the shape of a ring with cloud patterns. The obverse side is decorated with the sun, the moon, the star in charge of prosperity, and the Big Dipper while the reverse side is patterned with the Eight Diagrams. The bell has four small bronze balls in it, and could send out jingling sound when shaken to tell the folk the arrival of the medical practitioner.

Preserved in Shanghai Museum of Traditional Chinese Medicine

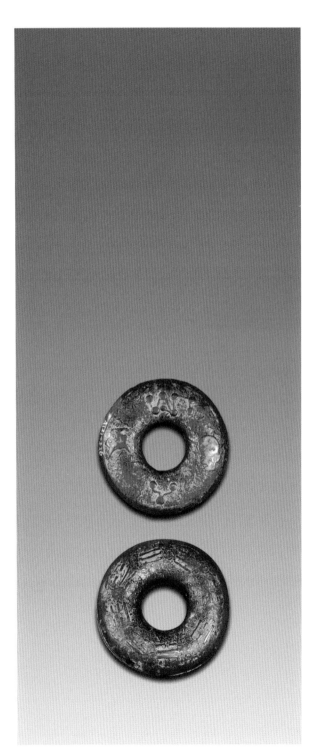

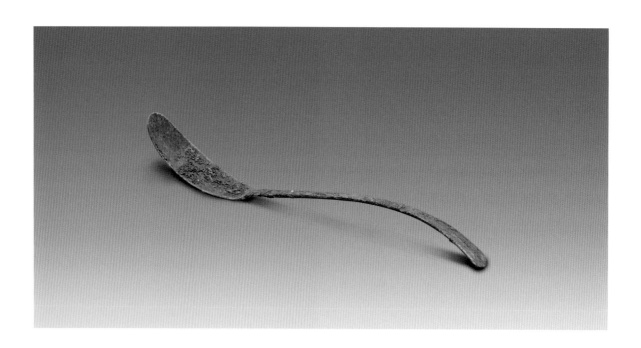

铜药匙

宋

铜质

长 22.6 厘米，宽 3.1 厘米，柄长 15 厘米

Bronze Medicine Spoon

Song Dynasty

Bronze

Length 22.6 cm/ Width 3.1cm/ Handle Length 15 cm

匙体扁平，中间内凹，柄较细长，呈弧形，尾部下弯。局部锈蚀较严重。四川省剑阁道教墓出土，同出土的丹瓶按道教方位排列，故应为炼丹用具。剑阁县文物管理所调拨。

成都中医药大学中医药传统文化博物馆藏

The body of the spoon is relatively flat with an indent in the middle, while its handle is long and recurved. Part of the spoon is heavily rusted. It was unearthed from a Taoist grave in Jiange County, Sichuan Province. Unearthed together with the spoon was an elixir bottle. In the grave, the bottle and the spoon were arranged in a special position which is meaningful according to Taoism. They are believed to be used for alchemy. It was allocated from Jiange County Administration Office of Cultural Relics.

Preserved in Museum of Traditional Chinese Medicine Culture, Chengdu University of Traditional Chinese Medicine

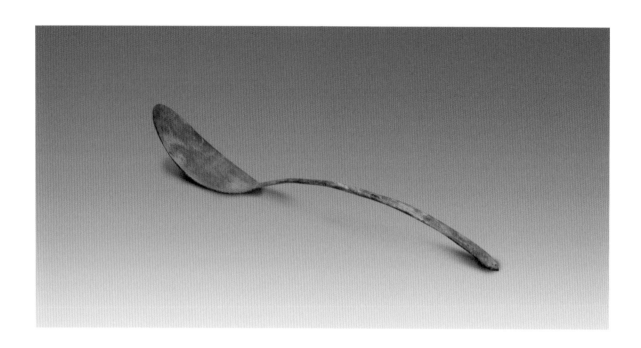

铜药匙

宋

铜质

长 22.4 厘米，宽 2.8 厘米，柄长 14.7 厘米

Bronze Medicine Spoon

Song Dynasty

Bronze

Length 22.4 cm/ Width 2.8 cm/ Handle Length 14.7 cm

匙体扁平，中间内凹，柄较细长，呈弧形，尾部下弯，器物锈蚀较严重，泛铜绿色。四川省剑阁道教墓出土，同出土的丹瓶按道教方法排列，故应为炼丹用具。剑阁县文物管理所调拨。

　成都中医药大学中医药传统文化博物馆藏

The body of the spoon is relatively flat with an indent in the middle, while its handle is long and recurved. The spoon is heavily rusted and looks aeruginous. It was unearthed from a Taoist grave in Chuangge County, Sichuan Province. Unearthed together with the spoon was an elixir bottle. In the grave, the bottle and the spoon were arranged in a special position which is meaningful according to Taoism. They are believed to be used for alchemy. It was allocated from Jiange County Administration Office of Cultural Relics.

Preserved in Museum of Traditional Chinese Medicine Culture, Chengdu University of Traditional Chinese Medicine

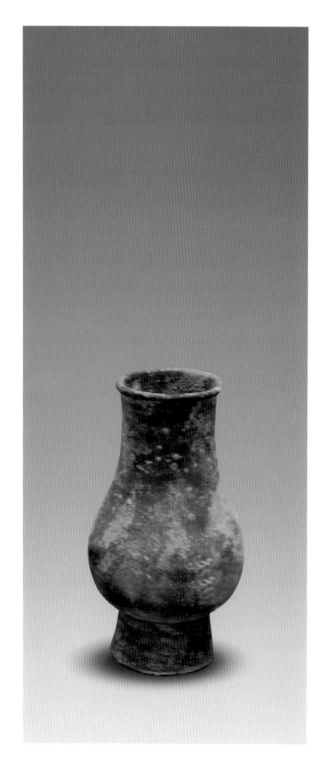

炼丹瓶

宋

铜质

口径 5.4 厘米，高 14 厘米

直颈，鼓腹，高圈足，表面有锈蚀痕迹，局部较严重，呈黑色。由剑阁县文物管理所调拨。

成都中医药大学中医药传统文化博物馆藏

Alchemy Bottle

Song Dynasty

Bronze

Mouth Diameter 5.4 cm/ Height 14 cm

The bottle has a straight neck, a bulged belly, and a tall ring foot. Part of it is heavily rusted and looks black. It was allocated from Jiange County Administration Office of Cultural Relics.

Preserved in Museum of Traditional Chinese Medicine Culture, Chengdu University of Traditional Chinese Medicine

炼丹瓶

宋

铜质

口直径 4.6 厘米，高 15.5 厘米

直颈，鼓腹，高圈足，表面锈蚀痕迹，呈铜绿色。
与道教的其他炼丹用具相伴出土。由剑阁县文物
管理所调拨。

成都中医药大学中医药传统文化博物馆藏

Alchemy Bottle

Song Dynasty

Bronze

Mouth Diameter 4.6 cm/ Height 15.5 cm

The bottle has a straight neck, a bulged belly, and a
tall ring foot. It is rusted and looks aeruginous. Along
with the bottle there were other unearthed tools for
Taoist alchemy. It was allocated from Jiange County
Administration Office of Cultural Relics.

Preserved in Museum of Traditional Chinese Medicine
Culture, Chengdu University of Traditional Chinese
Medicine

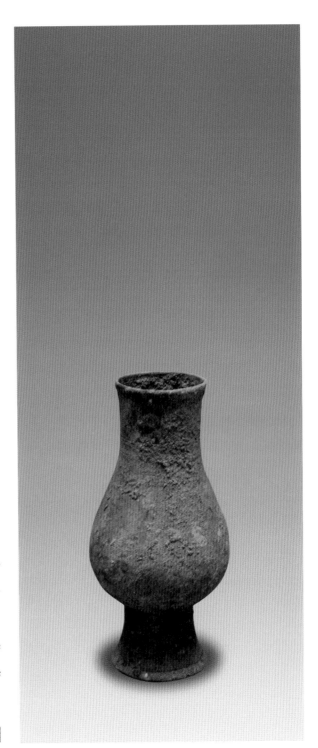

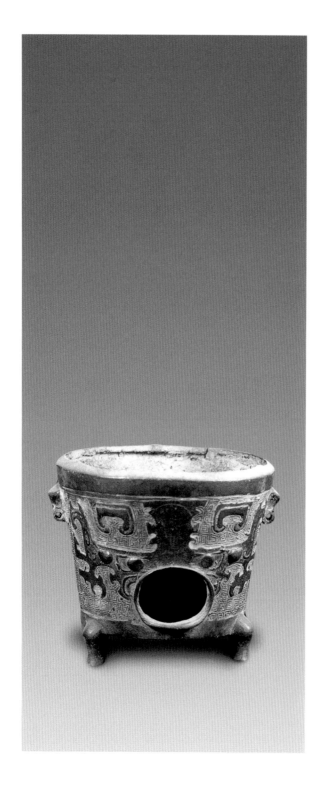

炼丹炉

宋

铜质

口径 15.5 厘米，底径 9.5 厘米，门阔 3.5 厘米，

高 21.5 厘米

Alchemy Furnace

Song Dynasty

Bronze

Mouth Diameter 15.5 cm/ Bottom Diameter 9.5 cm/

Fire Door Width 3.5 cm/ Height 21.5 cm

平面椭圆形。敞口，平底，三兽蹄形足，双耳，可系环。整器饰以雷纹，有凝重感。

上海中医药博物馆藏

The furnace is in the shape of a cylinder. Its orifice is spacious. It has a flat bottom and three beast-hoof-shaped feet. Its two ears are perforated. The furnace is decorated with thunder pattern which give a sense of dignity.

Preserved in Shanghai Museum of Traditional Chinese Medicine

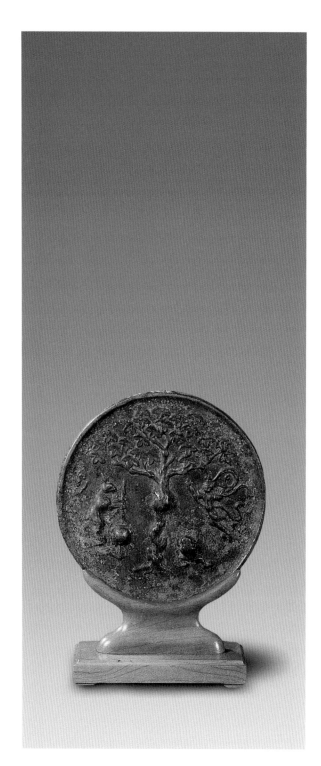

月宫玉兔捣药图铜镜

宋

铜质

直径 12 厘米

Mirror with the Moon Palace Motif

Song Dynasty

Bronze

Diameter 12 cm

圆形。镜背图案为玉兔捣药，桂树居中，左
为玉兔，右为嫦娥。

上海中医药博物馆藏

The mirror is round in shape. The picture on
its back consists of a rabbit crushing herbal
medicine on the left, a laurel tree in the middle,
and Chang'e on the right.
Preserved in Shanghai Museum of Traditional
Chinese Medicine

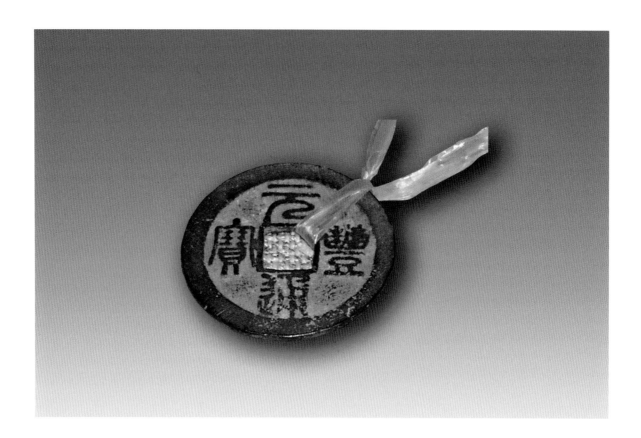

铜货币

宋

铜质

直径 2.8 厘米

Copper Currency

Song Dynasty

Copper

Diameter 2.8 cm

圆形钱，正面有"元丰通宝"字样，"元丰"
为宋神宗年号。货币。完整无损。陕西省历
史博物馆调拨。

陕西医史博物馆藏

This piece is a round currency with inscription
of "Yuan Feng Tong Bao" on its surface. Yuanfeng
is the title of Emperor Shenzong of Song(1078-
1085). It is intact and undamaged. It was
allocated from Shaanxi History Museum.

Preserved in Shaanxi Medical History Museum

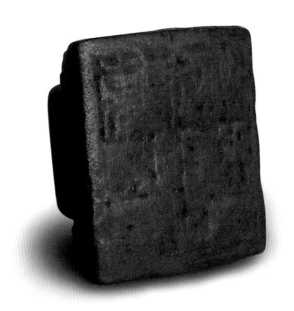

古酒务司印

宋

铜质

印面边长 4.3 厘米，高 4 厘米

Official Seal of Department in Charge of Alcohols

Song Dynasty

Bronze

Side Length 4.3 cm/ Height 4 cm

方形，直形钮。印面为篆体朱文。为公章。

严重磨损，字迹不清。

　中华医学会 / 上海中医药大学医史博物馆藏

The seal is square in shape with a straight handle. It was an official seal of a department in charge of alcohols. The characters carved on the seal are illegible because of severe wear.

Preserved in Chinese Medical Association/ Museum of Chinese Medicine, Shanghai University of Traditional Chinese Medicine

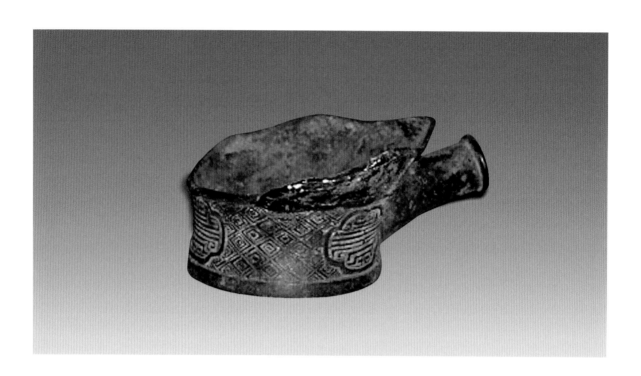

铜勺

宋

铜质

口径 9 厘米，底径 7 厘米，通高 5 厘米，重 200 克

口呈花瓣状，腹上饰云雷纹，中腹有一柄，平底。为生活器具。陕西省咸阳市征集。

陕西医史博物馆藏

Bronze Spoon

Song Dynasty

Bronze

Mouth Diameter 9 cm/ Bottom Diameter 7 cm/ Height 5 cm/ Weight 200 g

The orifice of the spoon is in the shape of a flower petal. Its belly is decorated with cloud and thunder patterns. The spoon has a handle in the middle of the belly and a flat bottom. It was collected in Xianyang City, Shaanxi Province.

Preserved in Shaanxi Museum of Medical History

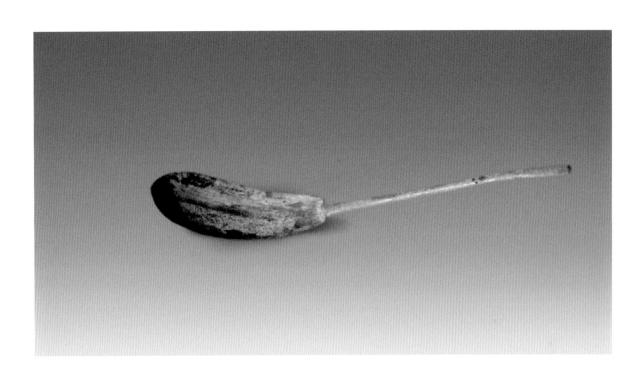

铜匙

宋

铜质

长 16.3 厘米 ， 匙身宽 2.6 厘米 ， 重 20 克

曲柄浅斗，状似今之羹匙。为食器。

广东中医药博物馆藏

Bronze Spoon

Song Dynasty

Bronze

Length 16.3 cm/ Width 2.6 cm/ Weight 20 g

The spoon is relatively flat and looks like the spoon we use today. It was used for eating.

Preserved in Guangdong Chinese Medicine Museum

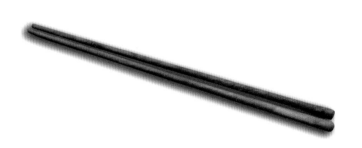

筷

宋

铜质

长 23 厘米

一对铜筷，细长圆柱形，一端大一端小，为食器。剑阁县文管所调拨。

成都中医药大学中医药传统文化博物馆藏

Chopsticks

Song Dynasty

Bronze

Length 23 cm

This pair of bronze chopsticks is slender and cylindrical in shape with one end bigger than the other. It was used for eating. It was allocated from Jiange County Administration office of Cultural Relics.

Preserved in Museum of Traditional Chinese Medicine Culture, Chengdu University of Traditional Chinese Medicine

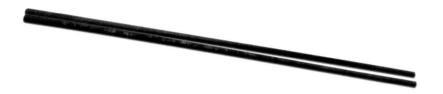

筷

宋

铜质

长 25 厘米

一对铜筷，细长圆柱形，一端大一端小，为食器。
剑阁县文管所调拨。

成都中医药大学中医药传统文化博物馆藏

Chopsticks

Song Dynasty

Bronze

Length 25 cm

This pair of bronze chopsticks is slender and
cylindrical in shape with one end bigger than the
other. It was used for eating. It was allocated from
Jiange County Administration office of Cultural
Relics.

Preserved in Museum of Traditional Chinese Medicine
Culture, Chengdu University of Traditional Chinese
Medicine

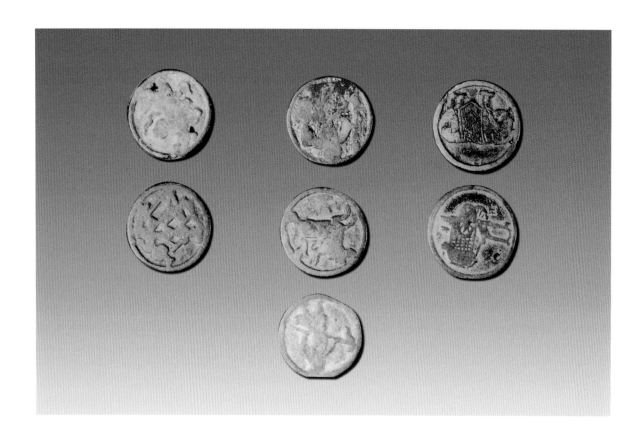

铜质象棋子

宋

铜质

直径 2~2.5 厘米

Bronze Chinese Chess Pieces

Song Dynasty

Bronze

Diameter 2−2.5 cm

象棋子为铜铸而成，共计 18 枚。除将子稍
大外，其余大小相若，两面皆铸成与象棋子
相应名字的图案。

中国体育博物馆藏

The collection consists of a total of 18 Chinese
chess pieces made of bronze. Two of them are
bigger than the others. There are corresponding
designs on both sides.

Preserved in China Sports Museum

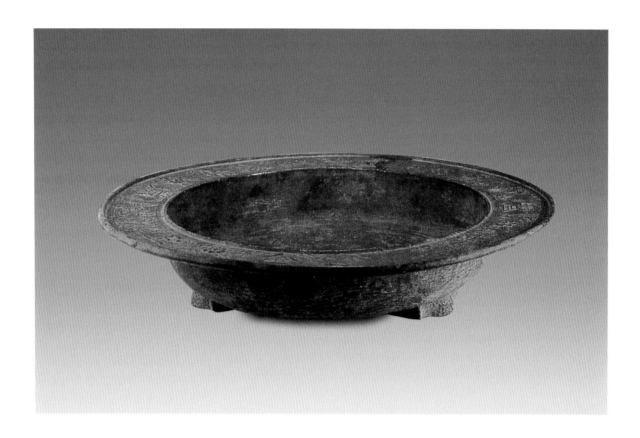

三鱼铜盆

宋

铜质

口沿外径 30.3 厘米，内径 21.4 厘米，底径 21 厘米，通高 5.7 厘米，足高 1.2 厘米

Bronze Basin

Song Dynasty

Bronze

Outer Diameter 30.3 cm/ Inner Diameter 21.4 cm/ Bottom Diameter 21 cm/ Height 5.7 cm/ Foot Height 1.2 cm

盆底中有牡丹纹，围有浮塑三鱼；盆沿饰花
草纹，有"金玉满堂，长命富贵"八字铭文。
是一件精美的盥洗器。陕西咸阳北塬出土。

陕西省医史博物馆藏

On the bottom of the basin, three raised fishes
in relief are swimming around a peony. The
rim with flower and grass designs is inscribed
with 8 characters which mean abundant wealth
and longevity with many children in the family.
The exquisite basin was used as a utensil
for washing. It was excavated in Beiyuan of
Xianyang City, Shaanxi Province.

Preserved in Shaanxi Museum of Medical History

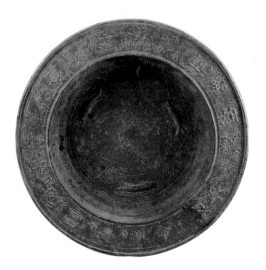

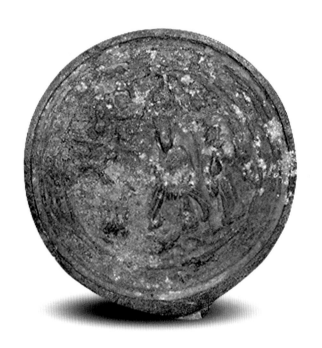

铜镜

宋

铜质

直径 10 厘米，重 100 克

圆形，镜中心为三瓣花图案。为生活器具。半残。

陕西医史博物馆藏

Bronze Mirror

Song Dynasty

Bronze

Diameter 10 cm/ Weight 100 g

The mirror is round in shape. The center of its back is decorated with a three-petaled flower. The mirror, an item for daily use, was partly damaged.

Preserved in Shaanxi Museum of Medical History

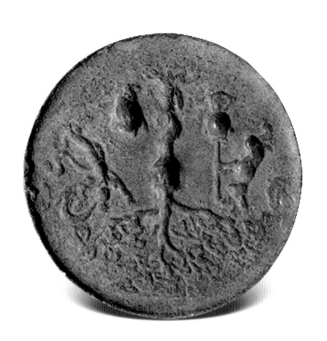

月宫嫦娥铜镜

宋

铜质

直径 12.4 厘米，厚 0.6 厘米，重 345 克

圆形。背面为月宫图，中为桂树，左为嫦娥，右

为玉兔捣药。

广东中医药博物馆

Bronze Mirror Patterned with Chang'e in the Moon Palace

Song Dynasty

Bronze

Diameter 12.4 cm/ Thickness 0.6 cm/ Weight 345 g

The mirror is round in shape. Its back is decorated with a picture of the Moon Palace with the goddess Chang'e on the left, a rabbit grinding medicinal herbs on the right and a laurel tree in the middle.

Preserved in Guangdong Chinese Medicine Museum

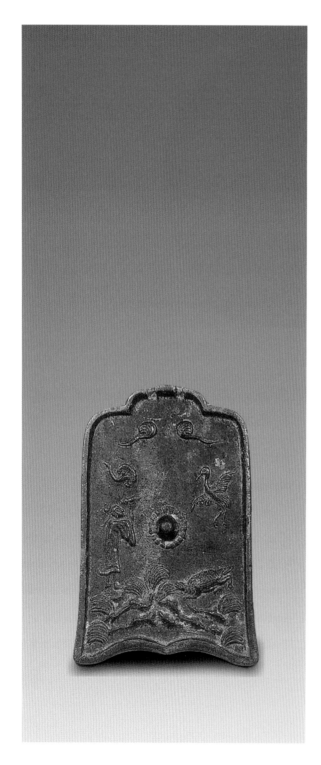

龟咽鹤息气功纹铜镜

宋

铜质

通高 12 厘米

Bronze Mirror with Qi Gong Scene

Song Dynasty

Bronze

Height 12 cm

钟形，圆钮。镜背图案的近景松林中，有一只正摇头伸颈呈吐气状的龟，右上角一只仙鹤在飞翔，左侧有一位直立拱手遥望着远处飞鹤的老者，正在做气功。这是一幅典型的"龟咽鹤息"式气功图。

湖南省博物馆藏

This mirror is shaped like a bell. Its knob is hemispherical. At the bottom of its back, a turtle in a pine forest is breathing with its neck extended, while a crane is flying in the sky at the top right corner. On the left side of the knob there is an old man practicing Qi Gong, breathing exercises. The scene is typical of one pattern of Qi Gong.

Preserved in Hunan Provincial Museum

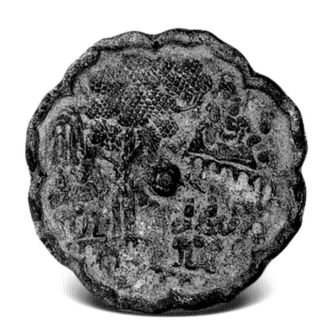

观棋人物纹铜镜

宋

铜质

直径 11.7 厘米

Bronze Mirror with Scene of Playing Chinese Chess

Song Dynasty

Bronze

Diameter 11.7 cm

八瓣菱花形。圆钮。钮右上部两人席地而坐

正在弈棋，中间一人观棋。钮下树两侧各有

二人姿态相同，身着短褐，双手弯曲上抬，

似边走边谈。

中国体育博物馆藏

The mirror is in the shape of a linghua flower
with eight petals. Its knob is hemispherical. At
the upper right part of the knob, two people are
sitting face to face, playing chess, with another
person standing in the middle and watching
them. Below the knob on each side of the tree,
two persons are walking side by side, chatting
with each other.

Preserved in China Sports Museum

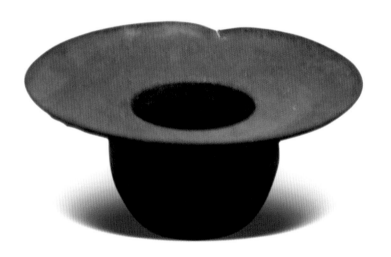

唾盂

宋

铜质

口径 20 厘米，高 48 厘米

Spittoon

Song Dynasty

Bronze

Diameter 20 cm/ Height 48 cm

圆盘状口，微残一缺口，口阔大且由外向内微微倾斜，便于使用。腹微鼓，平底，束颈。是较常见的漱口吐痰用具。器物造型规整，铜质较好，外部已锈成墨绿色。成都平原考古出土，1990 年由成都市博物馆调拨。

成都中医药大学中医药传统文化博物馆藏

The spittoon has a dish-shaped mouth with a gap, a bulged belly, a contracted neck, and a flat base. It was a common utensil for rinsing the mouth and spitting. The spittoon has a well-structured shape and quality bronze except for the dark green exterior due to rusting. The spittoon was unearthed in Chengdu Plain. It was allocated from Chengdu Museum, in 1990.

Preserved in Museum of Traditional Chinese Medicine Culture, Chengdu University of Traditional Chinese Medicine

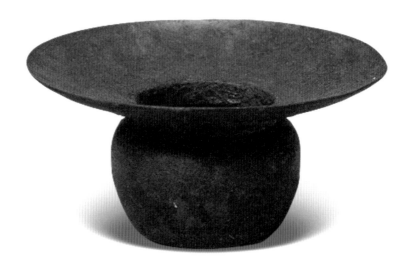

唾盂

宋

铜质

口径 20 厘米，高 8.4 厘米

Spittoon

Song Dynasty

Bronze

Mouth Diameter 20 cm/ Height 8.4 cm

圆盆状口，鼓腹，平底。是较常见的漱口
吐痰用具。表面锈蚀。

成都中医药大学中医药传统文化博物馆藏

The spittoon has a dish-shaped mouth, a
bulged belly, and a flat base. Its surface is
covered with rust. The spittoon was a common
utensil for rinsing the mouth and spitting.
Preserved in Museum of Traditional Chinese
Medicine Culture, Chengdu University of
Traditional Chinese Medicine

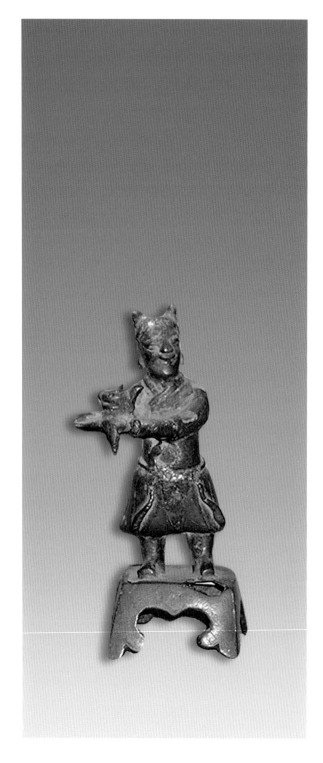

铜香童

宋

铜质

口径 2 厘米，底径 5.4 厘米，通高 12.2 厘米，
重 300 克

Bronze Figurine of Incense Boy

Song Dynasty

Bronze

Mouth Diameter 2 cm/ Bottom Diameter 5.4 cm/

Height 12.2 cm/ Weight 300 g

香童双手持一香炉，立于一四足底座上。为
礼器。底座有残。陕西省咸阳市征集。

陕西医史博物馆藏

This figurine is a boy holding an incense burner
and standing on an incomplete base with four
feet. The artifact was a sacrificial item. It was
collected in Xianyang City, Shaanxi Province.
Preserved in Shaanxi Museum of Medical History

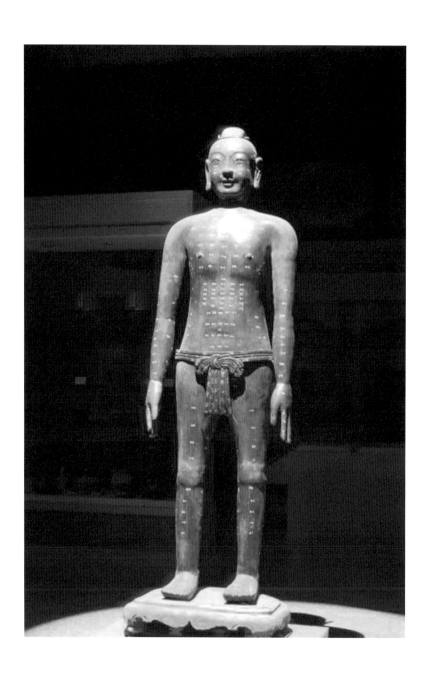

针灸铜人

宋

铜质

高 173 厘米

仿宋天圣针灸铜人。身高和青年男子相仿，面部俊朗，体格健美。头部有头发及发冠；上半身裸露，人形正立，两手平伸，掌心向前。铜人被浇铸为前后两部分，利用特制的插头来拆卸组合。铜人标有 354 个穴位，所有穴位都凿穿小孔。体腔内有木雕的五脏六腑和骨骼。宋天圣针灸铜人北宋天圣五年（1027）宋仁宗诏命翰林医官王惟一所制造。中国古代供针灸教学用的青铜浇铸而成的人体经络腧穴模型。

北京御生堂中医药博物馆藏

Acupuncture Bronze Figurine

Song Dynasty

Bronze

Height 173 cm

Tian Sheng acupuncture bronze figurine of Song style is close to a young and handsome adult in height and body building. The standing figurine is half naked with a bun on his hair and two hands stretching out naturally on both sides of his body. It is casted into two segments which are connected with a special plug. There are 354 acupuncture points on the body and each of them is carved with holes. The cavity of the body is carved with wooden internal organs and bones. Tian Sheng acupuncture bronze figurine was made by the imperial physician Wang Weiyi authorized by Emperor Ren Zong during the fifth years of Tian Sheng of the Northern Song Dynasty. The human body meridian model casted with bronze was used for acupuncture teaching in ancient China.

Preserved in Chinese Medicine Museum of Beijing Yu Sheng Tang Drugstore

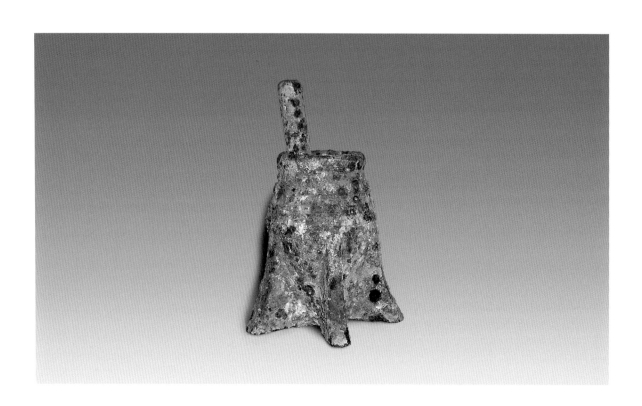

铁药臼

金

铁质

臼：口径 11.7 厘米，底径 27 厘米，通高 23.5 厘米，重 1170 克

铁杵：长 31 厘米，直径 3.1 厘米

Iron Mortar and Pestle

Jin Dynasty

Iron

Mortar: Mouth Diameter 11.7 mm/ Bottom Diameter 27 cm/ Height 23.5 cm/ Weight 1,170 g

Pestle: Length 31 cm/ Diameter 3.1 cm

臼为圆唇，折腹，蹼足。杵为圆柱形，一端为手柄，稍小；一端为捣药处，稍大。制药工具。陕西省澄城县善化乡征集。

陕西医史博物馆藏

The mortar has a round rim, a bugled belly, and web-shaped feet. The pestle is like a rod with one end slightly bigger than the other. The collection was used for pounding drugs. Both the mortar and the pestle were collected in Shanhua of Chengcheng County, Shaanxi Province.

Preserved in Shaanxi Museum of Medical History

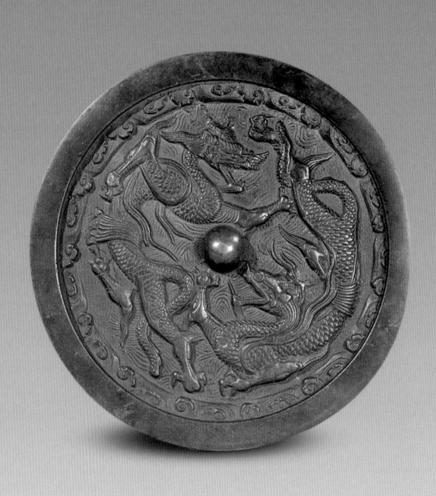

双龙纹镜

金

铜质

直径 22.2 厘米

圆形。圆钮。镜背凸铸双龙，张牙舞爪，首尾相接，呈追逐状。镜缘有"都右院"刻款及花押。"都右院"是金代常设的铜器检验机构。1952 年原东北文化局文物处移交。

辽宁省博物馆藏

Mirror with Design of Two Dragons

Jin Dynasty

Bronze

Diameter 22.2 cm

The mirror is circular in shape with a hemispherical knob. The back of the mirror has a design of two raised dragons chasing each other with baring fangs and brandishing claws. Characters of inscriptions indicating the bronze-inspecting body in the Jin Dynasty and signature are carved on the edge of the mirror. The mirror was transferred by Cultural Relics Division of former Northeastern Culture Bureau in 1952.

Preserved in Liaoning Provincial Museum

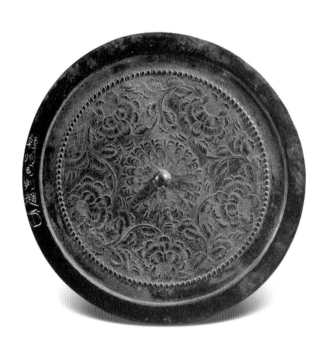

韩州司判牡丹纹镜

金

铜质

直径 21.3 厘米

Mirror with Peony Pattern

Jin Dynasty

Bronze

Diameter 21.3 cm

圆形。圆钮，菊花瓣钮座。主题纹饰为五朵缠枝牡丹花，花朵饱满，刻画细致入微。外圈饰以一周圆珠纹。镜缘刻铭及花押。此镜制作精良，在金镜中不可多得。1978 年吉林省梨树县出土。

吉林省博物院藏

The mirror is circular in shape with a hemispherical knob which sits on a chrysanthemum-shaped base. The principal motifs are composed of five plump peonies enclosed by a ring of pearl patterns. Characters of inscription and signature are carved on the edge of the mirror. This well-made mirror, which is rare for its exquisite workmanship among mirrors of the Jin Dynasty. It was unearthed in Lishu County, Jilin Province, in 1978.

Preserved in Jilin Provincial Museum

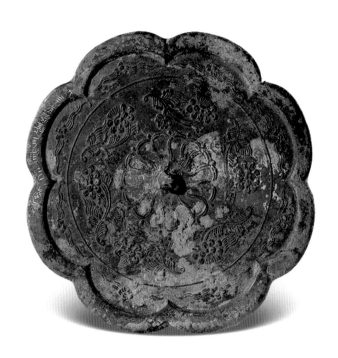

太原府录事司官葵花镜

金

铜质

直径 21.3 厘米

Mirror with Mallow Flower Designs

Jin Dynasty

Bronze

Diameter 21.3 cm

八瓣葵花形。圆钮，葵花形钮座。其外环饰
六株折枝牡丹花，外圈为流云纹。镜缘刻铭
及花押。1941 年山西省太原市出土。

中国国家博物馆藏

The mirror is in the shape of a mallow flower
with eight petals. Its hemispherical knob sits
on a mallow flower base. Its principal motifs
are six peonies surrounded by floating clouds.
Characters of inscription and signature are
carved on the edge. The mirror was unearthed
in Taiyuan City, Shanxi Province, in 1941.
Preserved in National Museum of China

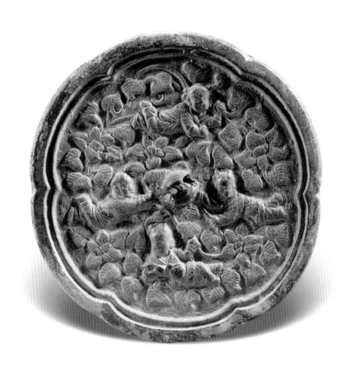

四童戏花葵花镜

金

铜质

直径 13.8 厘米

Mallow-shaped Mirror with the Design of Four Children

Jin Dynasty

Bronze

Diameter 13.8 cm

六瓣葵花形。圆钮。镜背满布花丛，四童子
躺卧其中，神态各异，或举手持花，或低头
赏花，憨态可掬。此镜纹饰用浮雕手法表现，
为金镜中的精品。1956年吉林省长春市出土。

吉林省博物院藏

The mirror is in the shape of a mallow flower
with six petals. The knob is hemispherical in
shape. The back of the mirror is decorated with
patterns of flower clusters and four charming
and naive boys lying among the flowers. These
children wear different postures: some are
holding flowers in their hands while others are
enjoying the flowers. All the patterns are in
relief. The exquisite mirror was unearthed in
Changchun City, Jilin Province, in 1956.
Preserved in Jilin Provincial Museum

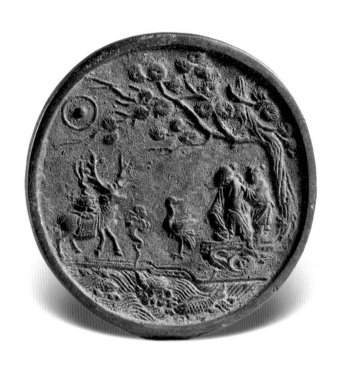

龟鹤人物镜

金

铜质

直径 13.3 厘米

Mirror with Designs of Figures, Crane and Turtle

Jin Dynasty

Bronze

Diameter 13.3 cm

圆形具柄镜，柄已失。镜背右侧斜生一松树，
树下石上站一老叟和一侍童。左上饰一轮红
日，其下一鹿驮着小儿缓缓而行。鹿前方有
灵芝一株，一仙鹤回首而望。下方波涛滚滚，
波中饰鱼、龟浮游。1983年吉林省榆树县（今
榆树市）出土。

榆树市博物馆藏

The mirror is circular in shape and its handle is
lost. The back of the mirror is decorated with
a scene. There is an oblique pine tree on the
right with an old man and his servant standing
under it. On the upper left, there is the rising
sun, under which a deer with a kid on its back is
walking slowly. In front of the deer are a glossy
ganoderma and a crane looking back. At the
bottom is a rolling river with fishes and turtles
swimming in it. The mirror was unearthed
in Yushu County (now Yushu City) , Jilin
Province, in 1983.

Preserved in Yushu Museum

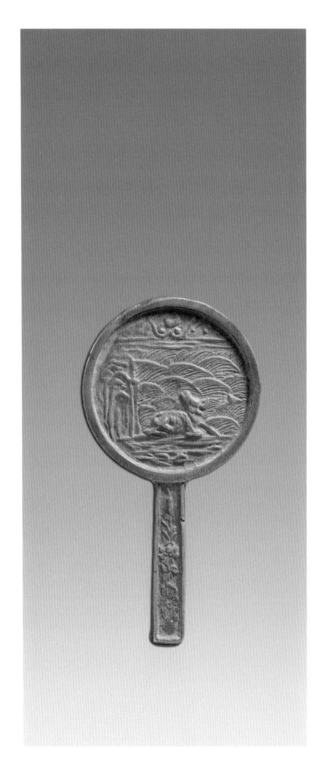

吴牛喘月纹柄镜

金

铜质

直径 8.5 厘米

Bronze Mirror with Scene of a Legend

Jin Dynasty

Bronze

Diameter 8.5 cm

圆形。长柄。镜背画面上方一轮明月从浮云中显现，下为翻滚的波涛。左侧岩石连着水中小洲，一牛卧于地上，回首望月。柄饰花叶纹。1987 年吉林省德惠县(今德惠市)出土。

长春市文物保护研究所藏

The mirror is circular in shape with a long handle decorated with patterns of flowers and leaves. The picture on its back illustrates a Chinese idiom about the buffaloes that mistook the moon for the hot sun. At the top of the picture a bright moon is emerging from the floating clouds. At the bottom is a rolling river. A buffalo is lying on the ground, looking up at the moon and panting heavily. On the left of the buffalo there is a rock connected with the islet. The handle of the mirror is decorated with floral patterns. The mirror was unearthed in Dehui County (now Dehui City) , Jilin Province, in 1987. Preserved in Changchun Municipal Institute of Cultural Relics Protection

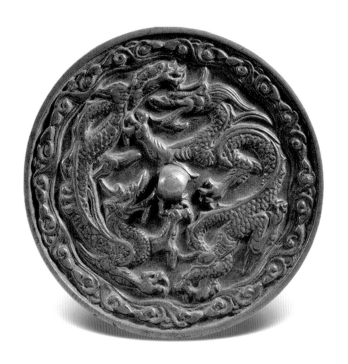

双龙纹镜

金

铜质

直径 18 厘米

Mirror Patterned with Two Dragons

Jin Dynasty

Bronze

Diameter 18 cm

圆形。圆钮。镜背双龙首尾相对而置，一龙躯体舒展，一龙弓身扭曲。双龙都有一后爪与龙尾相缠。外圈饰一周卷叶纹。镜缘刻"拿里虎千户"及花押。吉林省扶余市出土。

吉林省博物馆藏

The mirror is circular in shape with a hemispherical knob. The back of the mirror is patterned with two dragons, one with its body stretched and the other with its body twisted. Each dragon has one of its hind claws twined with its tail. The dragons are enclosed by a ring of rolled leaves. Five characters of inscription and signature are carved on the edge. The mirror was unearthed in Fuyu County, Jilin Province.

Preserved in Jilin Provincial Museum

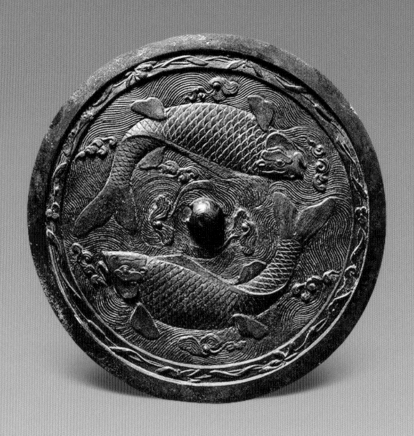

双鲤纹镜

金

铜质

直径 43.5 厘米

圆形。圆钮。钮外两条鲤鱼同向回游，鱼张口吐泡，目圆睁，鳞纹清晰，侧身摆尾，翻转自如，在碧波中逐浪嬉戏，形态逼真生动。镜背满布线条流畅细密的水波纹，波涛起伏的水面漂浮片片水草，显示出浓厚的自然情趣。1976 年黑龙江省阿城出土。

中国国家博物馆藏

Mirror Patterned with Two Carps

Jin Dynasty

Bronze

Diameter 43.5 cm

The mirror is circular in shape with a hemispherical knob. The principal motifs are two carps swimming in the same direction with open mouths, round eyes and distinct scales. They are swimming on their sides and wagging their tails to chase each other in the clear water. The designs, real, natural and vivid, are water ripples on which aquatic plants are floating. The mirror was unearthed in Acheng, Heilongjiang Province, in 1976.

Preserved in National Museum of China

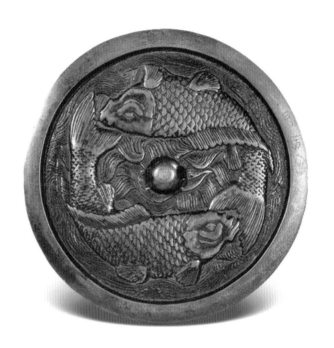

双鲤纹镜

金

铜质

直径 19.4 厘米

Mirror Patterned with Two Carps

Jin Dynasty

Bronze

Diameter 19.4 cm

圆形。圆钮。主题纹饰为两条浮雕的鲤鱼，首
尾相接，呈同向回游状。双鲤身躯肥硕，鳞、
鳍清晰，造型生动逼真。近缘处饰波纹一周，
边缘上刻"平州录事司官"及花押。

辽宁省博物馆藏

The mirror is circular in shape with a hemispherical
knob. The principal motifs are two big and fleshy
carps which are carved in relief with one's nose
connected with the other's tail and are chasing
each other. The outer region is decorated with
ripple patterns. Six characters of inscription and
signature are carved on the edge of the mirror.
Preserved in Liaoning Provincial Museum

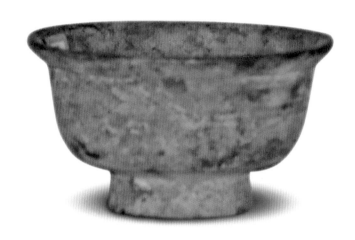

铜碗

元

铜质

口径 7.2 厘米，底径 3.4 厘米，通高 4 厘米，重 100 克

Bronze Bowl

Yuan Dynasty

Bronze

Mouth Diameter 7.2 cm/ Bottom Diameter 3.4 cm/ Height 4 cm/ Weight 100 g

敞口，直腹，圈足，中腹有一道棱。为食器。

碗底残。内蒙古自治区包头市征集。

陕西医史博物馆藏

This bowl has a flared mouth, a straight belly, and a ring foot. There is a ridge in the middle of its belly. The bottom is incomplete. The bowl was collected in Baotou City, Inner Mongolia Autonomous Region.

Preserved in Shaanxi Museum of Medical History

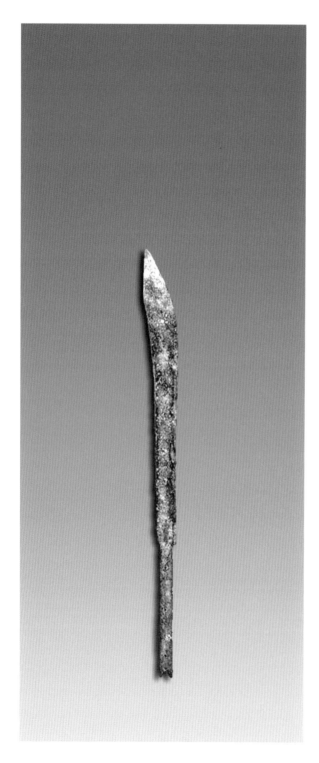

铁刀

元

铁质

长 80 厘米，宽 9.8 厘米

Iron Broadsword

Yuan Dynasty

Length 80 cm/ Width 9.8 cm

砍劈器械。扁条形刀柄，上有三穿，原应接长木柄；刀身后端匀直，前端稍宽，刀尖微上翘。此为元代蒙古族所用武术器械。

内蒙古博物院藏

The broadsword has been used for cutting or slashing. It has a flat strip-shaped hilt with three small holes, through which a long wooden handle ought to be connected. The rear end of the blade is perfectly straight, while the front end is slightly wider with an upturned tip. It is a martial arts weapon used by Mongolians of the Yuan Dynasty.

Preserved in Inner Mongolia Museum

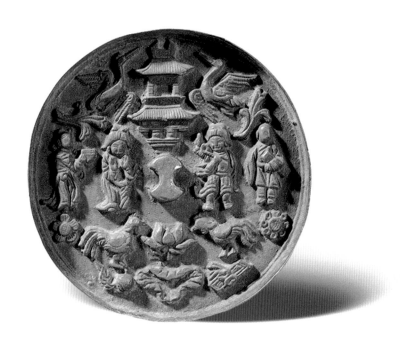

仙鹤人物镜

元

铜质

直径 9.7 厘米

Mirror with Patterns of Figures and Cranes

Yuan Dynasty

Bronze

Diameter 9.7 cm

圆形。元宝形钮。镜背画面共分三部分，上
饰阙楼和一对相向飞翔的仙鹤；中饰四名儿
童嬉戏；下饰一对公鸡，并间饰莲花和杂宝。
高棱镜边。河南省洛阳市孟津县朝阳镇出土。

洛阳博物馆藏

The mirror is circular in shape with an ingot-
shaped knob. The upper part of the mirror
back is decorated with two flying cranes and
a pavilion. In the middle part four children
are playing. In the lower part are two cocks
standing among lotus patterns. The edge of the
mirror is narrow and raised. The mirror was
unearthed in Chaoyang Town, Mengjin County,
Luoyang City, Henan Province.
Preserved in Luoyang Museum

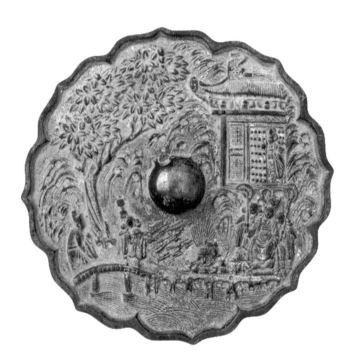

唐王游月宫鎏金菱花镜

元

铜质

直径 18.7 厘米

Linghua-shaped Gilt Mirror with the Moon Palace Scene

Yuan Dynasty

Bronze

Diameter 18.7 cm

八瓣菱花形。圆钮。通体鎏金。主题纹饰为月宫图。左

侧一株繁茂的桂树，右侧饰山门，门半掩，一人侧身远

眺，其旁有玉兔捣药。下侧为一桥，桥下波涛汹涌。桥

左侧一人，头戴官帽，弯腰拱手。桥右侧一人长袍束带，

坐于椅上，两侧各一执扇侍者。画面内容丰富，布局严

谨，反映了唐王游月宫的故事。1962 年宁夏回族自治

区隆德出土。

宁夏博物院藏

The gilt mirror is in the shape of a linghua flower with
eight petals. Its knob is hemispherical. The picture on the
back of the mirror is the Moon Palace. A flourishing laurel
tree stands on the left, while on the right there is the gate
to the palace with its door half open. A lady leans to her
side and looks far into the distance, and a rabbit nearby
is grinding herbs. At the bottom of the picture is a bridge
over a rolling river. On the left side of the bridge a person,
wearing an officer's hat, bends down with his hands to
his chest to salute. On the right side of the bridge, an
officer in a long robe sits in a chair with two servants on
his left and right sides fanning him. The picture, with rich
content and well-structured layout, depicts the story of the
emperor of the Tang Dynasty touring in the Moon Palace.
The mirror was unearthed in Longde County, Ningxia Hui
Autonomous Region, in 1962.

Preserved in Ningxia Museum

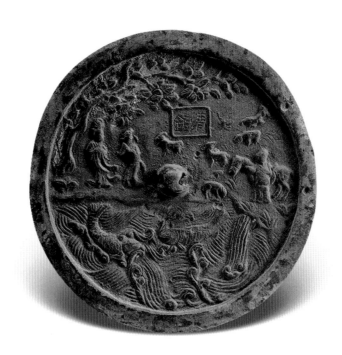

柳毅传书镜

元

铜质

直径 17.2 厘米

Mirror with the Scene of the Princess's Message

Yuan Dynasty

Bronze

Diameter 17.2 cm

圆形。圆钮。钮上方有"清铜"二字。镜背主题纹饰为民间传说的柳毅传书故事，左上方为一株枝叶繁茂的大树，一对男女在树下叙谈，书童牵马恭侍一旁。右上方为隐约的群山和飞鸟，羊儿在山中悠闲地吃草。下方是碧波涌动的湖水，鱼儿在水中嬉戏。此镜纹饰内容广泛，雕刻细腻，较为难得。1956 年湖南省长沙市征集。

湖南省博物馆藏

The mirror is round in shape with a hemispherical knob with two characters "Qing Tong" (bronze) above it . The scene on the back of the mirror depicts the folklore — "The Princess's Message". A man and a woman are chatting under a flourishing tree as a page boy waiting nearby with a horse. Birds are flying in the sky while sheep are grazing. At the bottom of the scene, there is a lake with fish swimming in it. The rich content of the patterns and delicate carving make the mirror precious. The mirror was collected in Changsha City, Hunan Province, in 1956.
Preserved in Hunan Provincial Museum

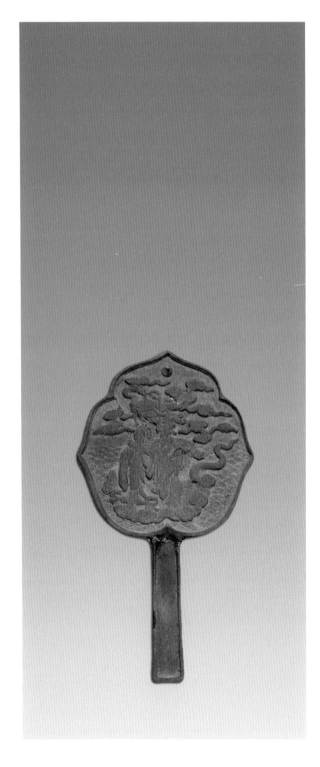

洛神菱花柄镜

元

铜质

直径 12.6 厘米

Linghua Flower Mirror Patterned with the Luo River Goddess

Yuan Dynasty

Bronze

Diameter 12.6 cm

三瓣菱花形。长柄。镜上方一轮明月，月光下，海浪中一童女手持华盖，一仙女亭亭玉立，若有所思。一童男双手捧物，仰望仙女。故事取材于《洛神赋》，为当时流行题材。1981 年吉林省九台区八家子村出土。

长春市文物保护研究所藏

The handled mirror is in the shape of a linghua flower with three petals. The Goddess of the Luo River is standing in the river under the moon with a maid nearby standing and holding a canopy. A page boy is looking up at the Goddess. The story came from *Ode to the Luo River Goddess*. The mirror was unearthed in Bajiazi Village, Jiutai District, Jilin Province, in 1981.

Preserved by Changchun Municipal Institute of Cultural Relics Protection

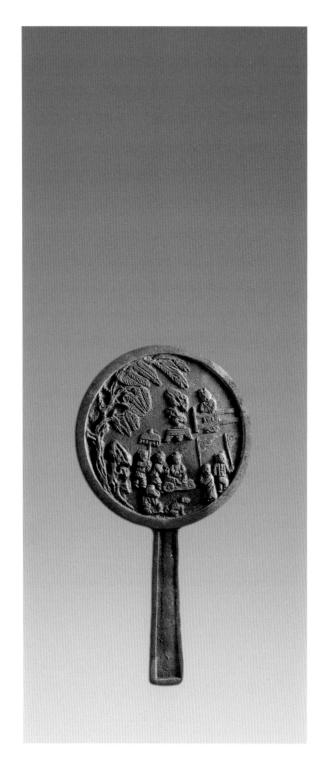

人物故事柄镜

元

铜质

直径 15.3 厘米

Bronze Mirror of a Story

Yuan Dynasty

Bronze

Diameter 15.3 cm

圆形。长柄。左侧置一树，树下一人手擎华盖，前有一人手推小车，车上坐一人。侧旁一人席地而坐，另有一卷尾小狗。前有两人手持三角旗开道，远处一妇人凭栏而望。树旁栏侧各置一块山石。1981年吉林省永吉县出土。

吉林省博物院藏

The mirror is round in shape with a long handle. On the left side is a tall tree under which a person is holding a canopy. In front of him another person is pushing a trolley with a child sitting in it. Another person is sitting on the ground not far away with a dog nearby. In the front, another two persons are holding burgees to clear the way. In the distance, a woman is standing on a bridge. The mirror was unearthed in Yongji County, Jilin Province, in 1981.

Preserved in Jilin Provincial Museum

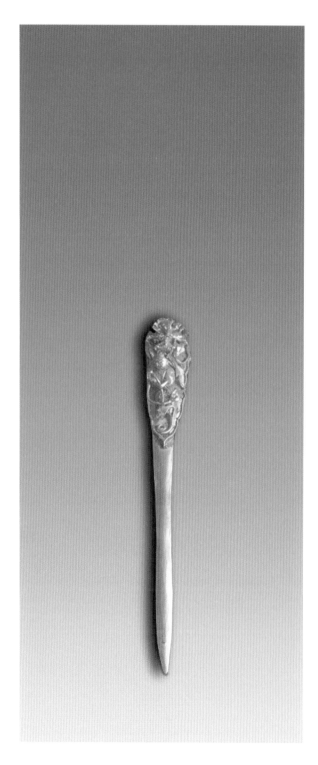

婴戏牡丹纹金簪

元

金质

长 13.4 厘米

Gold Hairpin with Peony Designs

Yuan Dynasty

Gold

Length 13.4 cm

簪体呈扁平状，簪头牡丹花叶繁盛，其间有一婴
孩手持一牡丹枝条正在玩耍，神态天真。婴戏牡
丹是我国古代工艺史上常用的装饰题材。金簪用
锤压、錾刻、焊接等工艺手法。南京市邓府山出土。

南京市博物馆藏

The hairpin is flat. The head of the hairpin is carved
with flourishing peony flowers and leaves, among
which a baby is playing with a peony branch. This
motif was a principal theme of decoration in ancient
China. Hammering, carving and welding skills
were used in making the hairpin. The hairpin was
unearthed from Mount Dengfu in Nanjing.

Preserved in Nanjing Municipal Museum

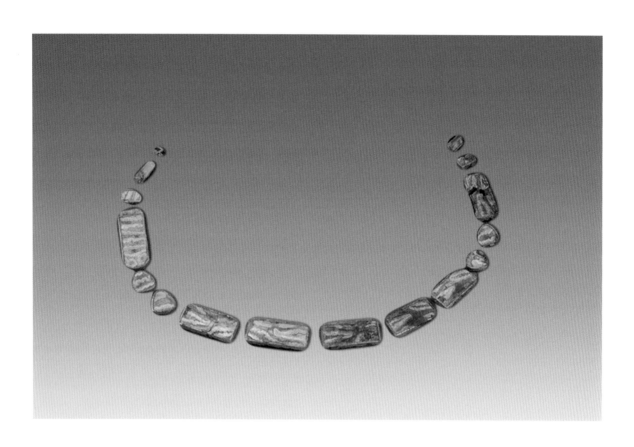

铜质鎏金镶孔雀石腰带

元

铜质

长 2.4~5.4 厘米，宽 2.2~2.4 厘米，厚 0.5 厘米

Gilt Bronze and Malachite Belt

Yuan Dynasty

Bronze

Length 2.4–5.4 cm/ Width 2.2–2.4 cm/ Thickness 0.5 cm

饰件计 15 块，其中长方形饰件 7 块，鸡心形饰件 4 块。其余尚有带头和带襻。带头的背面有 7 个小孔，呈梅花状。饰件的背后尚遗存有绸布布纹的痕迹，基本可认定，这些孔雀石饰件是镶嵌在蒙有绸布的皮革质腰带上的。这为研究南京及江南元代的丧葬习俗和服饰文化提供了实物资料。江宁区东山镇竹山公园出土。

江宁博物馆藏

The ornaments of the belt consist of 15 pieces, of which 7 are rectangular in shape, 4 are heart-shaped, and the other four are the belt buckle and ending pieces. There are 7 small holes shaped like a plum blossom on the back of the buckle. The malachite pieces are inlaid on the leather belt. The artifact provides physical information for studies on burial and costume customs in Nanjing and regions south of the Changjiang River of the Yuan Dynasty. The belt was unearthed in Jiangning District, Nanjing City. Preserved in Jiangning Museum

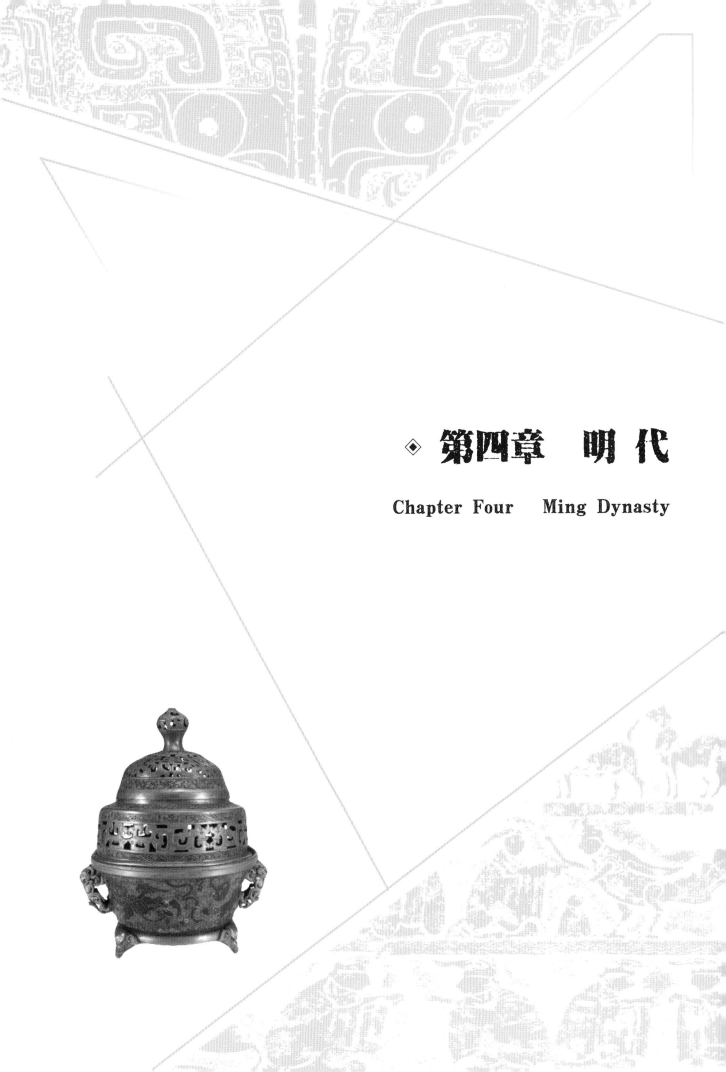

◆ 第四章 明 代

Chapter Four　Ming Dynasty

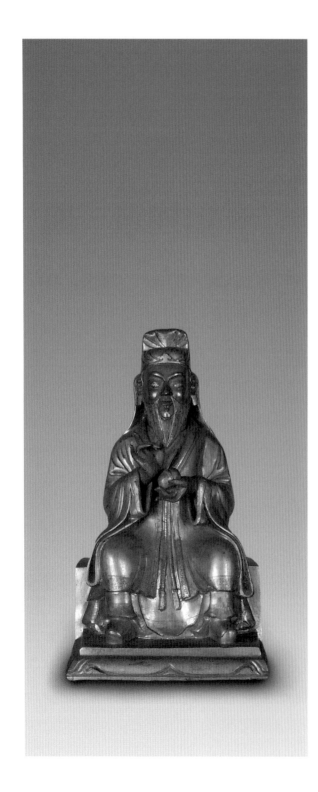

孙思邈像

明

铜质

宽 9.6 厘米，厚 7.9 厘米，通高 17.3 厘米

底面铜板：长 9.6 厘米，宽 7.9 厘米

Figurine of Sun Simiao

Ming Dynasty

Bronze

Width 9.6 cm/ Thickness 7.9 cm/ Height 17.3 cm

Base: Length 9.6 cm/ Width 7.9 cm

为唐代医家孙思邈安座太师椅全身像。坐像
底部铜板表面浅刻线条美观的道教图案，图
案中心是阴阳图，表面鎏金，工艺精湛。
1989 年入藏。

中华医学会 / 上海中医药大学医史博物馆藏

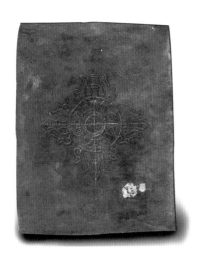

This full-length figurine is Sun Simiao, a
famous medical expert in the Tang Dynasty.
He sits quietly in an old-fashioned armchair.
The base of the statue is shallowly carved with
Taoist patterns with Yin and Yang designs in the
center. The gilt figurine, made with exquisite
workmanship, was collected in 1989.

Preserved in Chinese Medical Association/Museum
of Chinese Medicine, Shanghai University of
Traditional Chinese Medicine

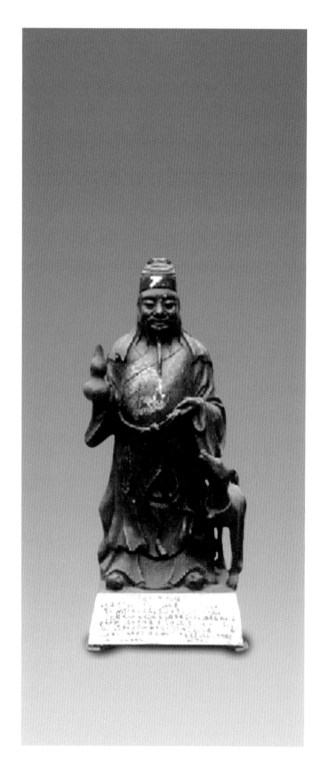

药圣韦慈藏塑像

明

铜质

高 27.8 厘米，重 2000 克

Bronze Figurine of Wei Cicang

Ming Dynasty

Bronze

Height 27.8 cm/ Weight 2,000 g

为药圣韦慈藏塑像，身着官服，手持葫芦，左侧立一犬。表面有彩绘，多已脱落。韦慈藏，唐代京兆人，曾官至光禄卿，后辞官深入民间，腰系葫芦，手牵黑犬，为民治病，疗疾神效，时人尊之为药圣，玄宗赐号药王。

广东中医药博物馆藏

This figurine is Wei Cicang, the medical sage. He is wearing an official's robe and holding a gourd in his right hand. A dog is standing at his left side. The surface of the statue was painted with colors, most of which have shredded. Wei Cicang, who was born in Chang'an (now Xi'an City), once was a high-ranking officer in charge of supplies in the palace. He resigned and then started his medical practice for common people. He was typically pictured as carrying a gourd and leading a black dog. Because of his miraculous curative effects, he was honored as a medical sage by the people of that time. Later he was rewarded with the title of the King of Medicine by Emperor Xuanzong of the Tang Dynasty.

Preserved in Guangdong Chinese Medicine Museum

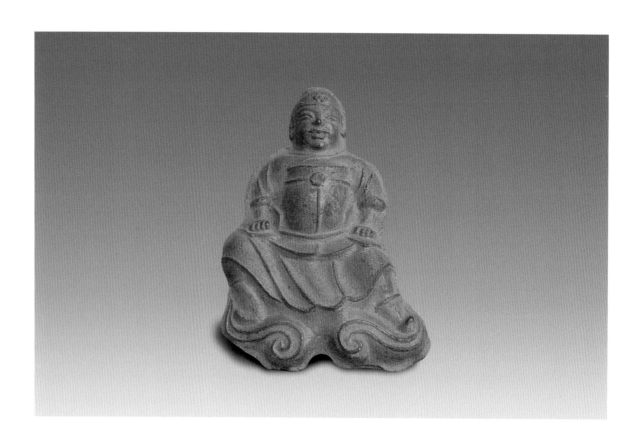

药王像

明

铁质

底径 14 厘米，高 20 厘米，头高 3.5 厘米，重 1900 克

Figurine of the King of Medicine

Ming Dynasty

Iron

Bottom Diameter 14 cm/ Height 20 cm/ Head Height 3.5 cm/ Weight 1,900 g

为药王塑像，坐状，足踩云，背较平，有两环。

陕西省延安市石佛洞遗物。

陕西医史博物馆藏

This sitting figurine is that of the King of Medicine in ancient China. It stands on clouds and its back is flat. It was discovered in Shifodong Cave in Yan'an City, Shaanxi Province.

Preserved in Shaanxi Museum of Medical History

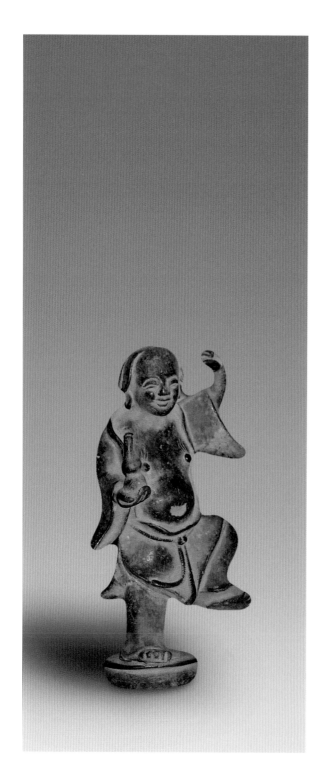

人物造像

明

铜质

通高 14 厘米，重 350 克

Figurine

Ming Dynasty

Bronze

Height 14 cm/ Weight 350 g

为宗教造像，人物袒胸露腹，神态生动。左
手举至头顶，右手捧一葫芦，左脚上跷，右
脚踩一圆盘底座。

陕西医史博物馆藏

The figurine, a religious statue, is bare chested
with lively postures. He is lifting his left hand
high above his head and holding a gourd in his
right hand. His left foot is lifted up and his right
foot is standing on a round disk-like base.
Preserved in Shaanxi Museum of Medical History

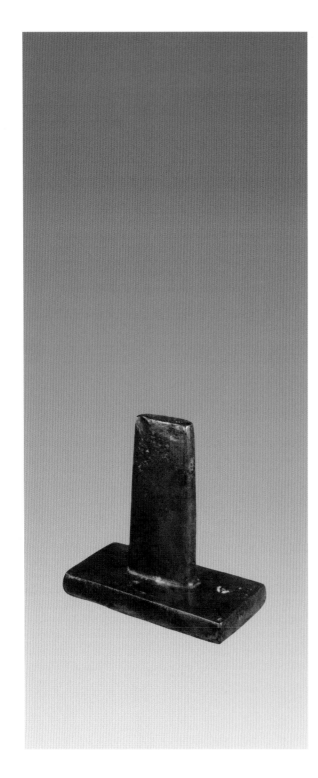

"高县医学记" 铜印

明

铜质

长 8.2 厘米，宽 4.2 厘米，把高 6.7 厘米

Bronze Seal of Medicine Department of Gao County

Ming Dynasty

Bronze

Length 8.2 cm/ Width 4.2 cm/ Handle Height 6.7 cm

明政府发给高县作为主管地方医学的钤记。印背左刻"高县医学记"，右边刻"礼部造洪武三十五年十二月日"字样。左图为其印蜕。

上海中医药博物馆藏

This was the official seal of a local department of medicine issued by the government of the Ming Dynasty. The characters carved on the left are the name of the local medicine department, while those carved on the right are the Ministry of Rites that had it made and the time when it was made. The picture on the left is the seal slough.

Preserved in Shanghai Museum of Traditional Chinese Medicine

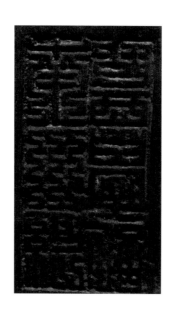

"南川县医学记"印

明

铜质

长 7.9 厘米，宽 4.2 厘米，通高 7.5 厘米

印文为九叠篆"南川县医学记"，其印背右侧刻
有同名字样，左上刻有"大顺二年四月日礼部造"，
印侧刻有"学字第三百三十一号"。为明末张献
忠时的县级医学印记。1951 年四川成都征集。

重庆博物馆藏

Bronze Seal

Ming Dynasty

Bronze

Height 7.5 cm/ Length 7.9 cm/ Width 4.2 cm

This was the official seal of a county medical
department in the Ming Dynasty. The characters
carved on it are the name of the medicine department,
the serial number of the seal, and the time when it
was issued by the Ministry of Rites in the Late
Ming Dynasty. The seal was collected in Chengdu,
Sichuan Province, in 1951.

Preserved in Chongqing Museum

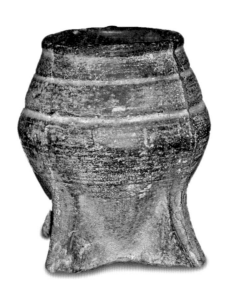

铁药臼

明
铁质
口径 11 厘米，底径 16 厘米，通高 17 厘米，重
4350 克
束口，圆唇，鼓腹，四棱底座，腹上有两圈弦纹。
捣碎药物用。

陕西医史博物馆藏

Iron Medicine Mortar

Ming Dynasty
Iron
Mouth Diameter 11 cm/ Bottom Diameter 16 cm/
Height 17 cm/ Weight 4,350 g
The mortar has a contracted mouth, a bulged belly,
and a base with four ridges. There are two raised
rings surrounding the belly. The mortar was used
for pounding medicinal herbs.
Preserved in Shaanxi Museum of Medical History

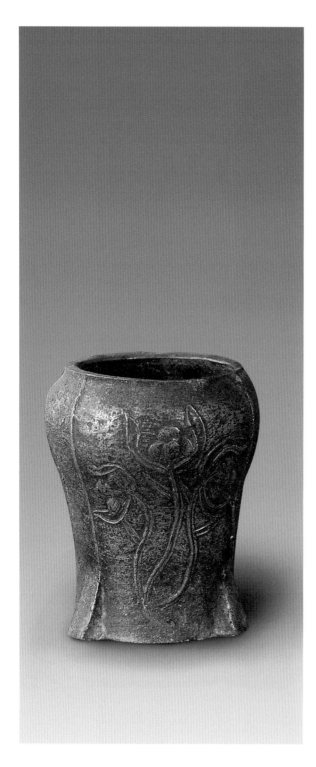

铜药臼

明

铜质

口径 10 厘米，高 14 厘米

Bronze Medicine Mortar

Ming Dynasty

Bronze

Mouth Diameter 10 cm/ Height 14 cm

束口，鼓腹，四棱底座。自口沿起至底足有三条直线，分开阳纹画面三幅，一为篆书长寿字，二为自山崖横出的黄芪，三为莲花。捣碎药物用。

上海中医药博物馆藏

The mortar has a contracted mouth, a bulged belly, and a base with four ridges. The mortar is decorated with three motifs. The first one is the Chinese seal character "Shou" (longevity), the second one is an atragalus growing out of the cliff, and the third one is a lotus. The mortar was used for pounding medicinal herbs.

Preserved in Shanghai Museum of Traditional Chinese Medicine

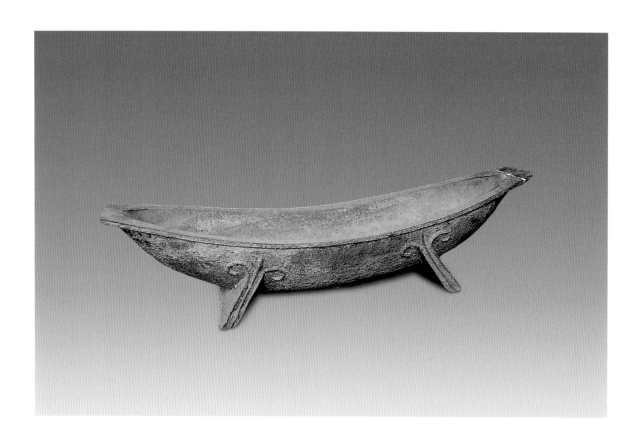

铁药碾

明

铁质

长 131 厘米，槽宽 25 厘米，高 23 厘米，重 100 千克

Iron Medicine Roller

Ming Dynasty

Iron

Length 131 cm/ Slot Width 25 cm/ Height 23 cm/ Weight 100 kg

略呈船形，中有凹槽，两板足，足上有环状纹，碾槽面两端各有"大吉"及"大利"的铭文。用于碾碎药物。

陕西医史博物馆藏

The roller is in the shape of a boat with a slot in the middle and two flat feet decorated with ring patterns. On both sides of the roller there are Chinese characters "Da Ji" (good luck) and "Da Li" (great fortune) as decorations. The roller was used for pulverizing medicinal herbs.

Preserved in Shaanxi Museum of Medical History

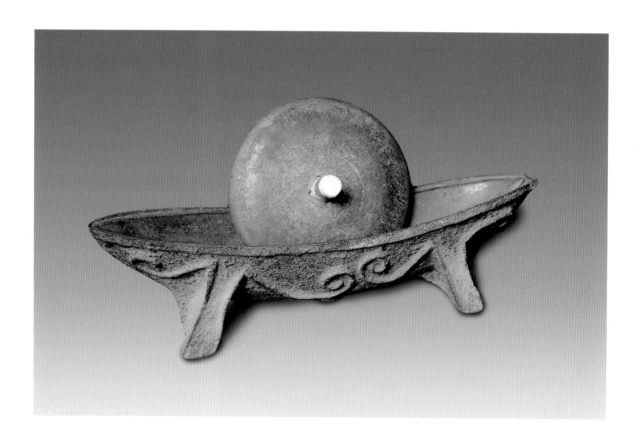

铁药碾

明

铁质

长 78 厘米，腹径 17 厘米，高 14 厘米，碾轮直径 30 厘米

Iron Medicine Roller

Ming Dynasty

Iron

Length 78 cm/ Belly Diameter 17 cm/ Height 14 cm/ Roller Wheel Diameter 30 cm

略呈船形，中有凹槽，两板足，一板足残。碾槽
两侧有卷云纹。抗日战争后期至解放战争时期曾
为青化砭保健药社所使用。

陕西医史博物馆藏

The roller is in the shape of a boat with a groove
in the middle and two flat feet, one of which is
damaged. Both sides of the roller are decorated with
curly clouds. It was used for pulverizing medicinal
herbs in Qinghuabian Clinic between the late period
of the War of Resistance Against Japan and the War
of Liberation.

Preserved in Shaanxi Museum of Medical History

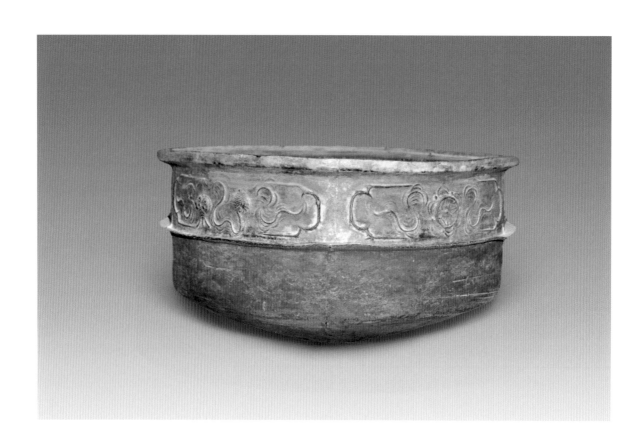

铜膏药锅

明

铜质

直径 48.5 厘米，通高 25 厘米

口沿上卷，折腹，圜底，底边上有浮雕图案。为
医药器具。

陕西医史博物馆藏

Bronze Plaster Pot

Ming Dynasty

Bronze

Diameter 48.5 cm/ Height 25 cm

The pot has a scrolled mouth rim, a twisted belly,
and a round base. It is decorated with patterns in
relief. The pot was used for pharmacy.

Preserved in Shaanxi Museum of Medical History

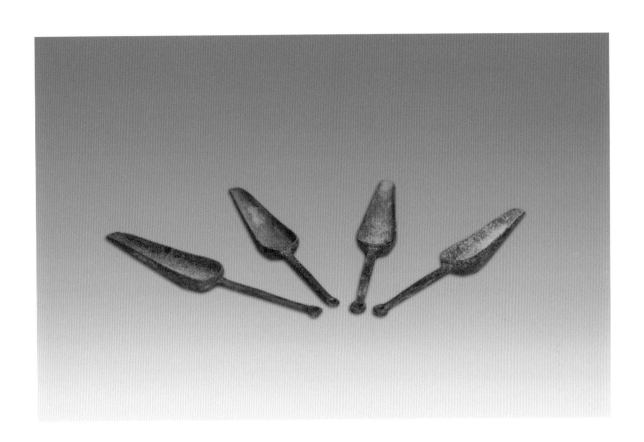

药勺

明

铜质

长 15 厘米，宽 2.5 厘米

勺行，长铲形，柄上刻有"天字号药匙"，柄端
为环首。为取药量具。

首都博物馆藏

Medicine Spoons

Ming Dynasty

Bronze

Length 15 cm/ Width 2.5 cm

These spade-shaped spoons have long handles on
which the names of their brand were carved. They
were used for measuring medicine.

Preserved in The Capital Museum

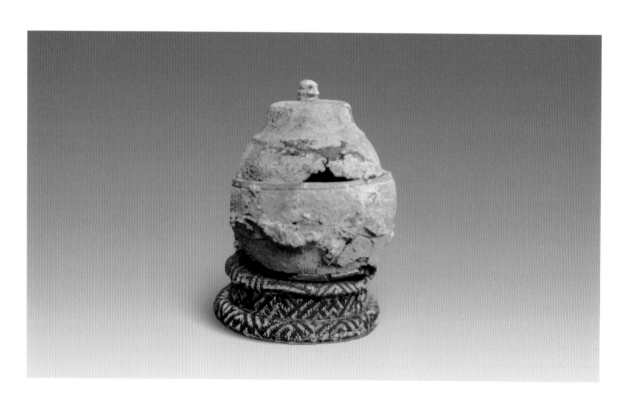

锡制盖罐两件并函

明

锡质

口外径 5.9 厘米，腹径 6.1 厘米，通高 6.53 厘米，腹深 3 厘米，重 135 克

平口，鼓腹下敛，平底，盖口与罐口相吻合，合成一罐状，盖顶宝珠钮。用于装置细药。

广东中医药博物馆藏

Tin Pot with a Lid

Ming Dynasty

Tin

Mouth Outer Diameter 5.9 cm/ Belly Diameter 6.1 cm/ Height 6.53 cm/ Belly Depth 3 cm/ Weight 135 g

The pot has a flat mouth rim, a round tapered belly, and a flat base. The lid which has a knob in the shape of a pearl, fits well with the mouth. It was a container for medicinal powders.

Preserved in Guangdong Chinese Medicine Museum

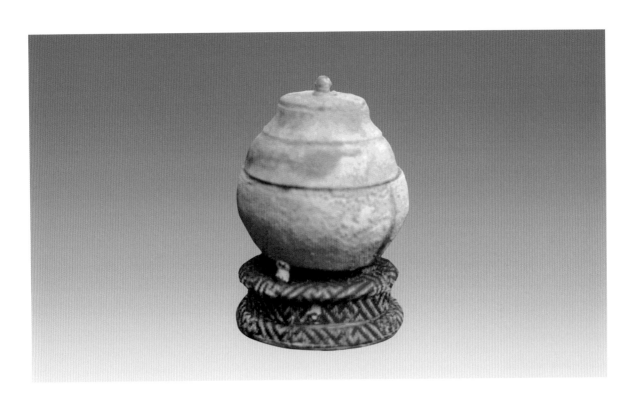

锡制盖罐两件并函

明

锡质

口外径 5.6 厘米，腹径 6 厘米，通高 7.15 厘米，
腹深 2.9 厘米，重 140 克

平口，鼓腹，下敛，平底，盖口与罐口相吻合，
合成一罐状，盖顶宝珠钮。用于装置细药。

广东中医药博物馆藏

Tin Jar with a Lid

Ming Dynasty

Tin

Mouth Diameter 5.6 cm/ Belly Diameter 6 cm/
Height 7.15 cm/ Belly Depth 2.9 cm/ Weight 140 g

The jar has a flat mouth rim, a round tapered belly,
and a flat base. The lid which has a knob in the
shape of a pearl, fits well with the mouth. It was a
container for medicinal powders.

Preserved in Guangdong Chinese Medicine Museum

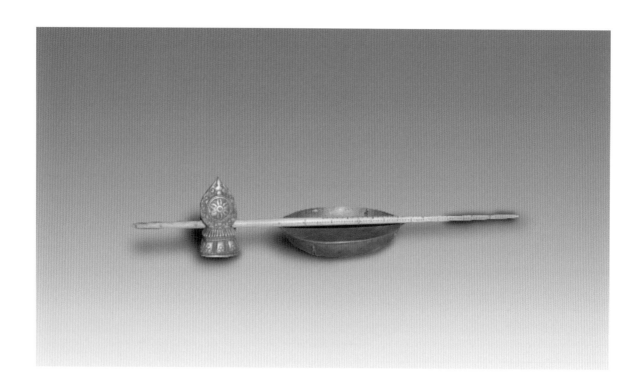

铜秤

明

铜质

杆长 30 厘米，砣高 5.7 厘米，盘口径 9 厘米，重 200 克

Bronze Steelyard

Ming Dynasty

Bronze

Steelyard Arm Length 30 cm/ Weight Height 5.7 cm/ Dish Diameter 9 cm/ Weight 200 g

由秤杆、秤砣和秤盘组成，盘和砣均有"万
历年制"的字样。为称量药物的器具。吴莲
芳征集。

陕西医史博物馆藏

The steelyard consists of an arm, a weight,
and a dish. Both the dish and the weight are
inscribed with words "Wan Li Nian Zhi",
meaning that it was made during Wanli Period
of the Ming Dynasty. The steelyard was used
for measuring medicinal herbs. It was collected
by Wu Lianfang.

Preserved in Shaanxi Museum of Medical History

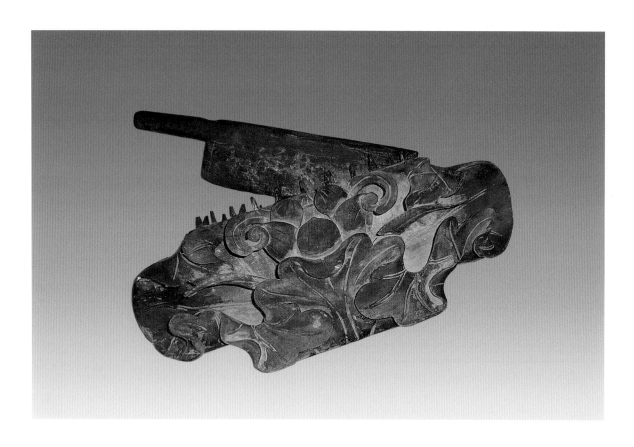

草药铡刀

明

铁质

长 44.5 厘米，宽 21 厘米

Medicinal Herb Chopper

Ming Dynasty

Iron

Length 44.5 cm/ Width 21 cm

草药铡由底槽和刀体组成，底槽呈云朵形，其上浮雕花叶纹，槽口有齿。刀体宽而锋利，一端连接底槽，一端装柄。中医药材加工的基础工具，在古代已广泛使用。一般小型制药作坊所使用的草药铡刀做工简单，形制单调。而此件草药铡刀，工艺精湛，风格粗犷，从纹饰和工艺上判断应属明代早期较大药房所私用。

张雅宗藏

The chopper is made up of a groove and a knife. The groove has a cloud shape decorated with flower and leaf patterns in relief and a dented notch. The knife's broad and sharp body is connected with the groove on one end and a handle on the other. The chopper was a basic tool widely used for Chinese medicinal material processing in ancient time. Medicinal herb choppers used in small drug-making mills have simple workmanship and single design. This artifact, however, shows exquisite craftsmanship and unconstrained style. Judging by its decorations and workmanship, this chopper is supposed to have been used privately in large pharmacies in early Ming Dynasty.

Collected by Zhang Yazong

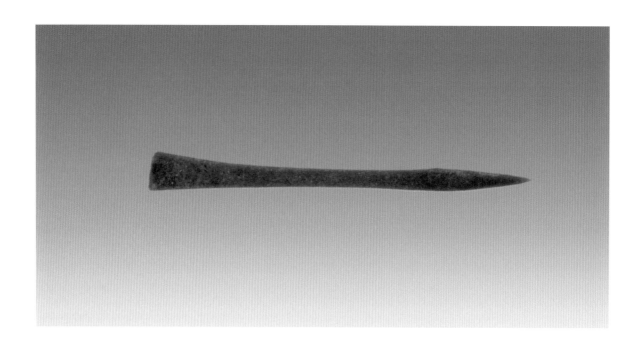

外科手术刀

明

铁质

长 16.7 厘米

柳叶形。一端为柄，一端有尖刃口，与现代手术刀相似。江苏省江阴夏颧墓出土。

江阴博物馆藏

Scalpel

Ming Dynasty

Iron

Length 16.7 cm

The scalpel is in the shape of a willow leaf. One end of it is the handle and the other end is the blade. The scalpel is similar to those used today. The knife was unearthed from Xia Quan's tomb in Jiangyin City, Jiangsu Province.

Preserved in Jiangyin Museum

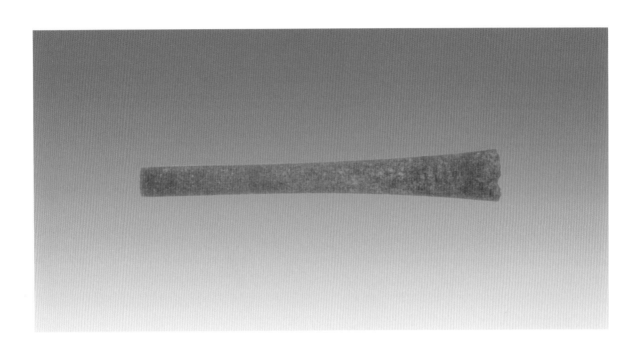

外科手术刀

明

铁质

长 11.3 厘米

长条形，一端为柄，另一端平刃。江苏省江阴夏
颧墓出土。

江阴博物馆藏

Scalpel

Ming Dynasty

Iron

Length 11.3 cm

This elongated knife has a long handle at one end
and a flat blade at the other. It was unearthed from
Xia Quan's tomb in Jiangyin City, Jiangsu Province.
Preserved in Jiangyin Museum

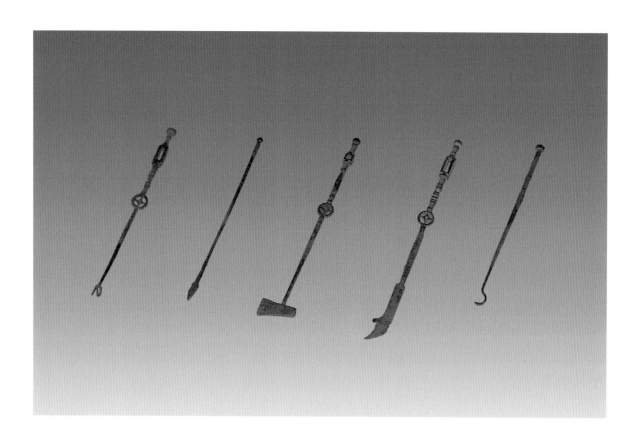

外科器具

明

铁质

Surgical Kit

Ming Dynasty

Iron

一套五件，包括斧、杈、烙铁、刀、弯钩刀。

均为民间医生用具。陕西省泾阳市征集。

陕西医史博物馆藏

This kit is composed of five surgical instruments:
an axe, a fork, a soldering iron, a knife, and
a hook knife, all of which were used by folk
doctors. The kit was collected from Jingyang
County, Shaanxi Province.

Preserved in Shaanxi Museum of Medical History

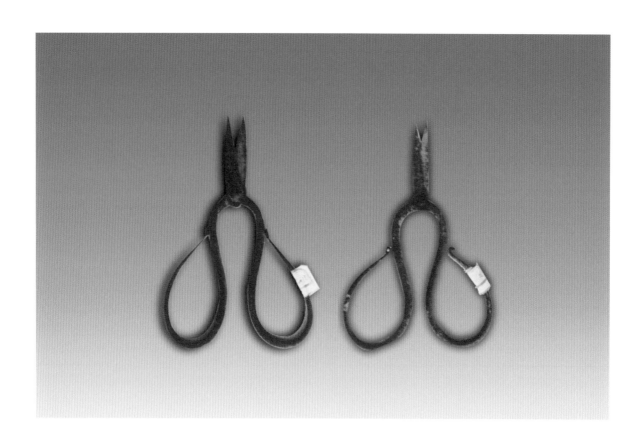

铁剪刀

Iron Scissors

明

Ming Dynasty

铁质

Iron

左：长 10.6 厘米

Left side: Length 10.6 cm

右：长 11.8 厘米

Right side: Length 11.8 cm

剪刀两把，形状与现代剪刀相似，均用于外

科手术器械。江苏省江阴夏颧墓出土。

江阴博物馆藏

The two pairs of scissors are similar to the scissors

we use today. They were surgical instruments. The

scissors were unearthed from Xia Quan's tomb in

Jiangyin City, Jiangsu Province.

Preserved in Jiangyin Museum

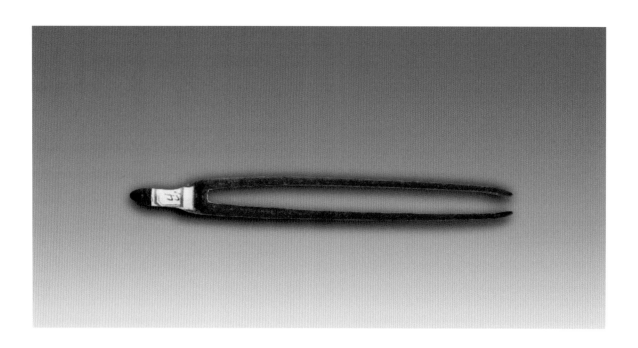

镊子

明

铁质

长 12.3 厘米

Tweezers

Ming Dynasty

Iron

Length 12.3 cm

一端为短柄，镊身细长，末端较尖。为外科
手术器械。江苏省江阴夏颧墓出土。

江阴博物馆藏

The pair of tweezers is long, thin and sharp-
pointed, with one end as a short handle. The
surgical instrument was unearthed from Xia
Quan's tomb in Jiangyin City, Jiangsu Province.
Preserved in Jiangyin Museum

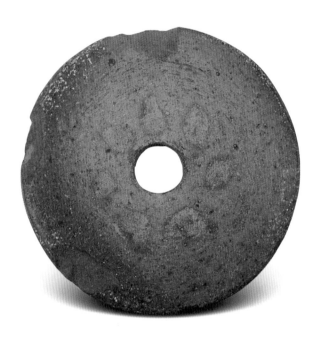

药碾轮

明

铁质

直径 13.9 厘米，厚 1.5 厘米

Drug-grinding Wheel

Ming Dynasty

Iron

Diameter 13.9 cm/ Thickness 1.5 cm

圆形，扁平状，中部有穿孔，孔周围有花瓣形纹饰。为制药流程中的磨制器具。中间孔洞应该配以与之相合的木棒，在研磨时用脚蹬踩木棒，使之在条形研磨池中上下移动，以达到磨碎药品的功能。

张雅宗藏

In the middle of the round and flat wheel there is a hole surrounded by petal patterns. The wheel was a grinding device used in drug preparation. The hole is supposed to work together with a wooden stick. A foot pedaled on the stick during grinding so that the stick could move upward and downward in the bar-shaped groove to grind drugs.

Collected by Zhang Yazong

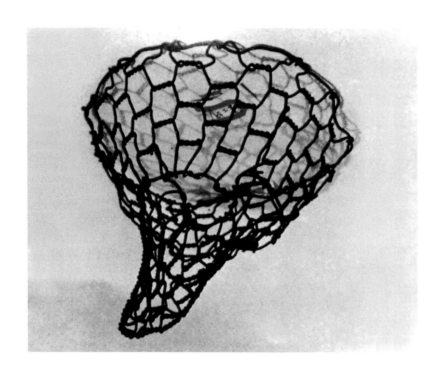

疝气托

明

铁质

罩口直径 11.5 厘米，高 11.5 厘米，重 51.4 克

Hernia Support

Ming Dynasty

Iron

Mouth Diameter 11.5 cm/ Height 11.5 cm/ Weight 51.4 g

系一圆锥形银丝罩，作用与现代疝气托同。此托放置于男尸大腿骨和盆骨之间，可知死者生前患有疝气。1974 年 4 月江苏省江阴夏颧墓出土。

江阴博物馆藏

This conical support was woven with silver wires. It has the same function as the hernia support we use today. This support was found to be placed between the deceased's thigh and pelvis, which indicates that this person had hernia when he was alive. The collection was unearthed from Xia Quan's tomb in Jiangyin City, Jiangsu Province, in April 1974.

Preserved in Jiangyin Museum

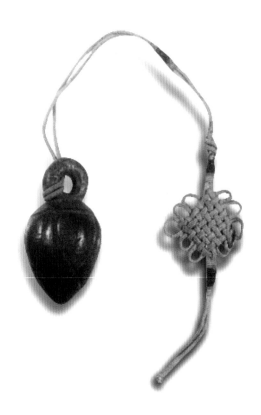

铜猎鞭锤

明

铜质

高 6 厘米，重 250 克

Bronze Whipping Hammer

Ming Dynasty

Bronze

Height 6 cm/ Weight 250 g

近似桃形，为一种技击器械，底部有环，可以系长链，便于技击。为古代武术器械中锤的一种。

中国体育博物馆藏

This artifact resembles a peach with a ring at its base, which can be tied to a long chain. It was one type of hammers used in martial arts in ancient time.

Preserved in China Sports Museum

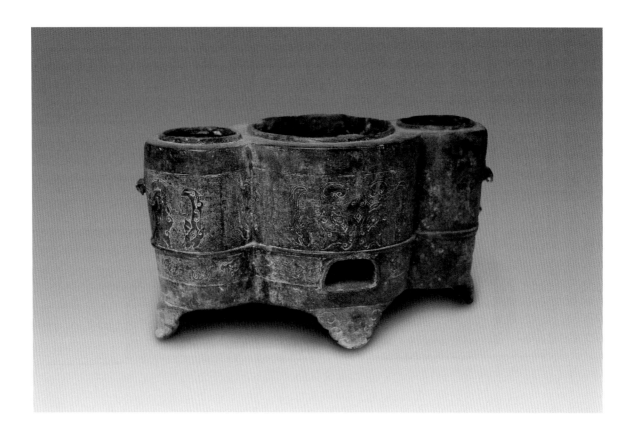

药炉

明

铜质

长 40 厘米，宽 22 厘米，高 21 厘米

Medicine Furnace

Ming Dynasty

Bronze

Length 40 cm/ Width 22 cm/ Height 21 cm

主炉堂由中空的双层壁及双层底组成，两旁
各有一个小炉膛通过主炉堂的夹壁及夹层底
相通，起到隔热、保温的作用。为明万历年
间太医院所用。

中国国家博物馆藏

The main part of the furnace consists of two
layers of walls and bases, which are connected
to the chambers on both sides. This structure
is effective for thermal insulation. This artifact
was the instrument used by the imperial hospital
in Wanli Period of the Ming Dynasty.

Preserved in National Museum of China

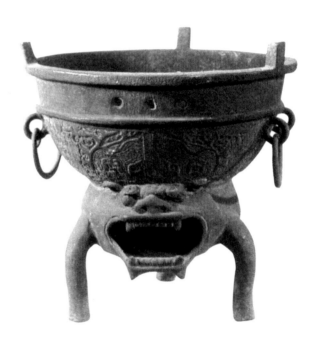

铜药炉

明

铜质

口径 28 厘米，高 32 厘米

Bronze Medicine Furnace

Ming Dynasty

Bronze

Mouth Diameter 28 cm/ Height 32 cm

敞口，深腹，三立足，双耳吊环，器表有兽
面纹。为制药工具。

上海中医药博物馆藏

The furnace has a flared mouth, a deep belly,
and three feet. There are two rings attached
to its belly. The surface is decorated with a
beast-face design. The furnace was used for
pharmacy.
Preserved in Shanghai Museum of Traditional
Chinese Medicine

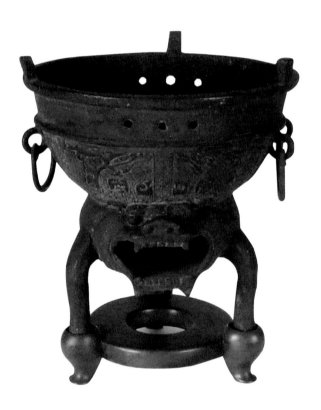

药炉

明

铁质

口外径 22.6 厘米，口内径 20.6 厘米，通高 22.3 厘米，风口 7.2 厘米 ×3.4 厘米，足高 7 厘米

Medicine Furnace

Ming Dynasty

Iron

Mouth Outer Diameter 22.6 cm/ Inner Mouth Diameter 20.6 cm/ Height 22.3 cm/ Fire Door Size 7.2 cm ×3.4 cm/

Foot Height 7 cm

炉状，敞口，深腹，柱状足，兽嘴形风口，炉身有套环拉手，口沿下有前后方各有三个小孔，表面有纹饰。为制药工具。1959年入藏。

中华医学会 / 上海中医药大学医史博物馆藏

The furnace has a flared mouth, a deep belly, three columnar feet, and a fire door shaped like a beast's mouth. There are two lantern rings attached to its belly and three small holes below the rim of the mouth in the front and at the back. The furnace was decorated with designs and was used for pharmacy. It was collected in 1959.

Preserved in Chinese Medical Association/ Museum of Chinese Medicine, Shanghai University of Traditional Chinese Medicine

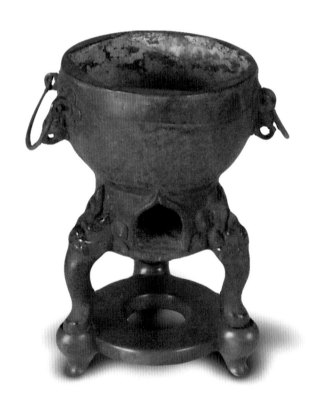

药炉

明

铁质

口外径 15.5 厘米，通高 21.2 厘米，风口 3.9 厘米 ×3.7 厘米

Medicine Furnace

Ming Dynasty

Iron

Mouth Outer Diameter 15.5 cm/ Height 21.2 cm/ Fire Door Size 3.9 cm ×3.7 cm

炉状，敞口，深腹，炉身有套环拉手，三兽脚足，兽嘴形风口，造型美观，表面有纹饰。为制药工具。1954 年入藏。

中华医学会 / 上海中医药大学医史博物馆藏

The furnace has a flared mouth, a deep belly, and three feet in the shape of beast's legs. There are two lantern rings attached to its belly. Its fire door resembles a beast's mouth. The furnace was used for pharmacy. It was collected in 1954.

Preserved in Chinese Medical Association/ Museum of Chinese Medicine, Shanghai University of Traditional Chinese Medicine

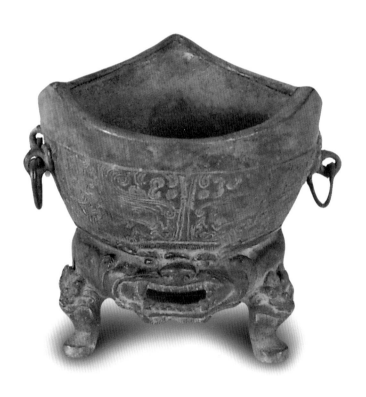

药炉

明

铁质

口径 16.7 厘米，通高 16.8 厘米

Medicine Furnace

Ming Dynasty

Iron

Diameter 16.7 cm/ Height 16.8 cm

炉状，敞口，炉身有套环拉手，三兽脚足，兽嘴形风口，口沿壁呈三个山峰状凸起。表面有纹饰。为制药工具。1959 年入藏。

中华医学会 / 上海中医药大学医史博物馆藏

The furnace has a flared mouth, three feet in the shape of beast legs, and a deep belly to which two lantern rings are attached. Its fire door resembles a beast's face. On the mouth there are three convexes. The surface of the furnace is decorated with designs. The furnace was collected in 1959.

Preserved in Chinese Medical Association/ Museum of Chinese Medicine, Shanghai University of Traditional Chinese Medicine

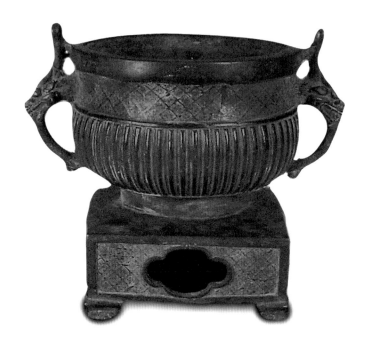

药炉

明

铁质

口外径 18.1 厘米，口内径 16.5 厘米，通高 23.8 厘米，风口 6 厘米 ×3.9 厘米

Medicine Furnace

Ming Dynasty

Iron

Mouth Outer Diameter 18.1 cm/ Mouth Inner Diameter 16.5 cm/ Height 23.8 cm/ Size of Fire Door 6 cm×3.9 cm

呈簋形，敞口，鼓腹，方座，炉身表面饰瓜纹，
有兽形双耳，椭圆花卉形风口，造型美观。
为制药工具。1959 年入藏。

中华医学会 / 上海中医药大学医史博物馆藏

The furnace resembles a round-mouthed food
vessel called gui with a flared mouth, a bulged
belly and a square bottom. The body surface is
decorated with melon designs. Two handles are
in the shape of a beast. The fire door is made
in the shape of an oval flower. The furnace was
used for pharmacy. It was collected in 1959.
Preserved in Chinese Medical Association/
Museum of Chinese Medicine, Shanghai
University of Traditional Chinese Medicine

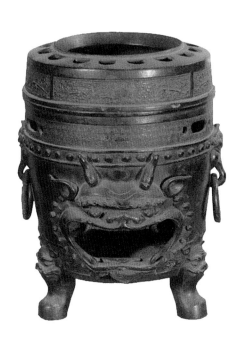

铜炼丹炉

明

铁质

口径 14 厘米，腹径 18 厘米，高 37 厘米

Bronze Alchemy Furnace

Ming Dynasty

Iron

Mouth Diameter 14 cm/ Belly Diameter 18 cm/ Height 37 cm

炉状，敛口，直腹，平底，双耳垂环，三兽
蹄形足。器表上部饰以云雷纹，中有一圈乳
丁纹，下饰兽面纹。为炼制丹药的炉具。

上海中医药博物馆藏

The furnace, which is shape like a cylinder,
has a contracted mouth, a straight belly, a flat
bottom, two dangling rings, and three paw-
shaped feet. The furnace is decorated with
cloud and thunder patterns in the upper part, a
ring of nipple pattern in the middle, and beast's
face patterns in the lower part. It was used for
alchemy.

Preserved in Shanghai Museum of Traditional
Chinese Medicine

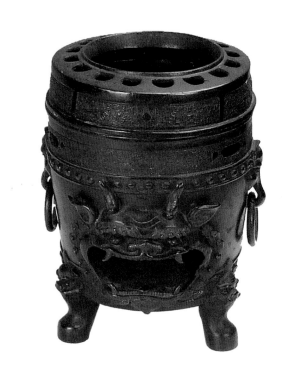

炼丹炉

明

铁质

口径 14.6 厘米，通高 29.5 厘米，足高 5.5 厘米，风口径 11.7 厘米 ×3.7 厘米

Alchemy Furnace

Ming Dynasty

Iron

Mouth Diameter 14.6 cm/ Height 29.5 cm/ Foot Height 5.5 cm/ Fire Door Size 11.7 cm ×3.7 cm

炉状，敛口，直腹，平底，双耳垂环，三兽蹄形足。正面有兽面纹，风口为兽嘴形，口沿上有多孔套圈。表面有纹饰精美，工艺精湛，光泽乌亮，造型优美。为炼制丹药的炉具。

中华医学会 / 上海中医药大学医史博物馆藏

The furnace, which is shaped like a cylinder, has a contracted mouth, a straight belly, a flat bottom, two dangling rings, and three paw-shaped feet. The front of the furnace is decorated with a beast's face pattern. Its fire door resembles a beast's mouth with a porous ferrule. The furnace has exquisite designs and ornaments, and looks jet-black. It was used for alchemy.

Preserved in Chinese Medical Association/ Museum of Chinese Medicine, Shanghai University of Traditional Chinese Medicine

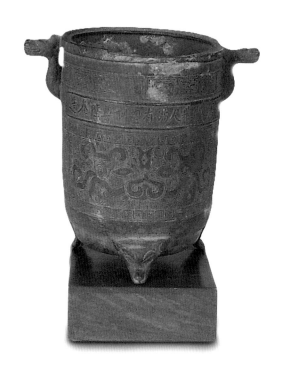

炼丹炉

明

铁质

口外径 15.9 厘米，口内径 13.2 厘米，通高 9.7 厘米，足高 1 厘米

Alchemy Furnace

Ming Dynasty

Iron

Mouth Outer Diameter 15.9 cm/ Mouth Inner Diameter 13.2 cm/ Height 9.7 cm/ Foot Height 1 cm

炉状，直口，直腹，平底，双兽形耳，三尖足。炉口有兽首钮，表面有纹饰，底面有"万历甲寅举人汤有望训导陆养造"字样。为炼制丹药的炉具。1959 年入藏。

中华医学会 / 上海中医药大学医史博物馆藏

The furnace, which is shaped like a cylinder, has a vertical mouth, a vertical belly, a flat bottom, and three pointed feet. It has two handles in the shape of a beast's head. Its surface is decorated with ornamentations and its bottom is carved with Chinese characters indicating the year when it was made and who made it. It was used for alchemy. The furnace was collected in 1959. Preserved in Chinese Medical Association/ Museum of Chinese Medicine, Shanghai University of Traditional Chinese Medicine

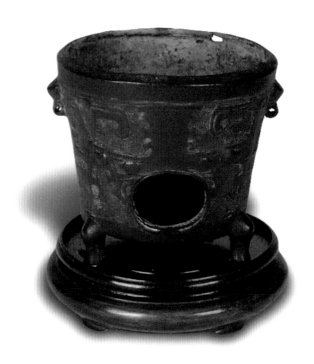

炼丹炉

明

铁质

口外径 12 厘米，通高 11.5 厘米，足高 1.7 厘米，风口径 4.1 厘米 ×3 厘米

Alchemy Furnace

Ming Dynasty

Iron

Mouth Outer Diameter 12 cm/ Height 11.5 cm/ Foot Height 1.7 cm/ Fire Door Size 4.1 cm ×3 cm

炉状，敞口，斜腹，平底，双耳，三兽蹄形足，椭圆形风口。表面饰兽纹、回纹。为炼制丹药的炉具。1959 年入藏。

中华医学会 / 上海中医药大学医史博物馆藏

The furnace, which is shaped like a cylinder, has a flared mouth, a beveled belly, a flat bottom, two ring handles, and three paw-shaped feet. Its fire door is oval in shape. The surface of the furnace is decorated with beast and fret patterns. It was used for alchemy. The furnace was collected in 1959.

Preserved in Chinese Medical Association/ Museum of Chinese Medicine, Shanghai University of Traditional Chinese Medicine

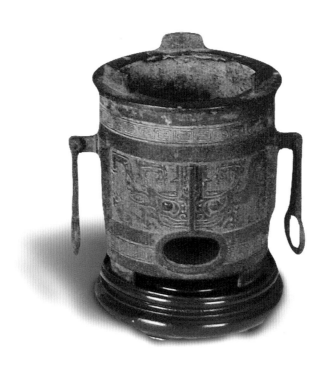

炼丹炉

明

铁质

口外径 14.7 厘米，口内径 10.9 厘米，通高 16 厘米，足高 1.3 厘米，风口径 4.3 厘米 ×2.3 厘米，

耳长 9.5 厘米

Alchemy Furnace

Ming Dynasty

Iron

Mouth Outer Diameter 14.7 cm/ Mouth Inner Diameter 10.9 cm/ Height 16 cm/ Foot Height 1.3 cm/ Fire Door

Size 4.3 cm×2.3 cm/ Handle Length 9.5 cm

炉状，直口，直腹，平底，折叠式双耳，三
扁平足，椭圆形风口，炉口有兽首钮，表面
饰兽面纹。为炼制丹药的炉具。1958 年入藏。

中华医学会 / 上海中医药大学医史博物馆藏

The furnace, which is shaped like a cylinder,
has a vertical mouth, a vertical belly, a flat
bottom, two folding handles, and three flat feet.
Its fire door is oval. The surface of the furnace
is decorated with beast's face patterns. It was
used for alchemy. The furnace was collected in
1958.

Preserved in Chinese Medical Association/
Museum of Chinese Medicine, Shanghai
University of Traditional Chinese Medicine

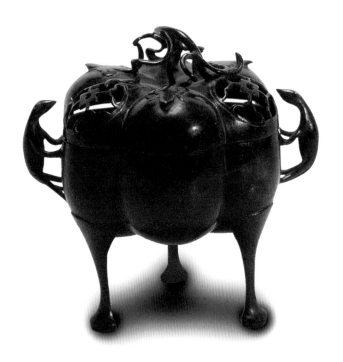

熏炉

明

铜质

腹径 10 厘米，高 14.5 厘米

Incense Burner

Ming Dynasty

Bronze

Belly Diameter 10 cm/ Height 14.5 cm

六瓣瓜棱形，上方有圆形镂孔三个，顶部以植
物枝茎虬屈代替把手，两侧壁塑有壁虎状动物
作为耳，下部三足支撑。

　　成都中医药大学中医药传统文化博物馆藏

The burner resembles a melon with six segments.
There are three holes in its lid. The knob of its lid
was is in the shape of plant stems. The handles on
both sides are in the shape of a lizard. The burner
has three feet.

Preserved in Museum of Traditional Chinese
Medicine Culture, Chengdu University of
Traditional Chinese Medicine

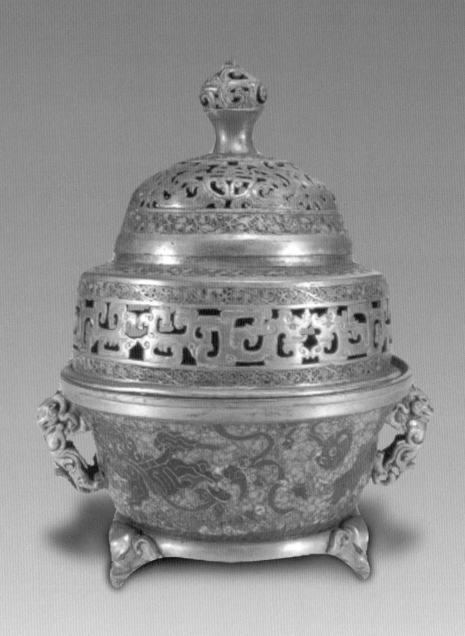

铜镀金掐丝珐琅双耳熏炉

明

铜质

口径 19 厘米，高 28 厘米，足径 14 厘米

炉体铜胎镀金，圆身，双兽耳，三象首足，镂空夔凤捧寿双层盖，龙钮。炉身通体以浅蓝釉为地，腹部饰掐丝珐琅双狮戏球花纹。

故宫博物院藏

Gilt Incense Burner

Ming Dynasty

Bronze

Mouth Diameter 19 cm/ Height 28 cm/ Foot Diameter 14 cm

This incense burner has a round belly, two beast-shaped handles, and three feet in the shape of an elephant's head. Its lid has two layers with a dragon knob and hollowed-out dragon and phoenix designs. The whole burner is covered with light-blue glaze, and wiry enamel craft was employed to decorate its body with two lions playing a ball.

Preserved in The Palace Museum

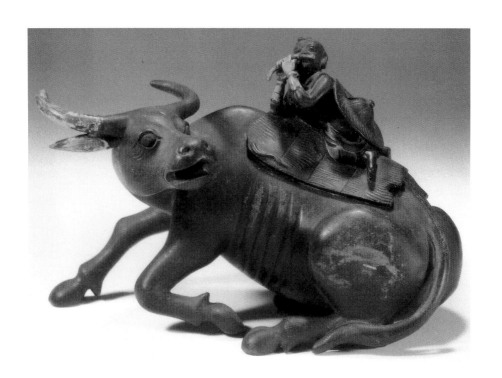

牧童骑牛形铜熏炉

明

铜质

通高 14 厘米

Bronze Incense Burner Patterned with a Cowboy on Buffalo

Ming Dynasty

Bronze

Height 14 cm

牛呈半卧状，回首，长尾下垂。器的腹部中空，
用于贮存香料。背顶有一长方形盖，盖钮铸
一牧童骑在牛背之上，身背带孔草帽，短笛
横吹，悠然自得。

河北博物院藏

The buffalo, in a semi-reclining position, is
looking back with a drooping tail. The hollow
space in its belly is the incense container. The
lid on the back of the buffalo is rectangular
with a knob in the shape of a cowboy wearing a
straw hat and playing the flute leisurely.
Preserved in Hebei Museum

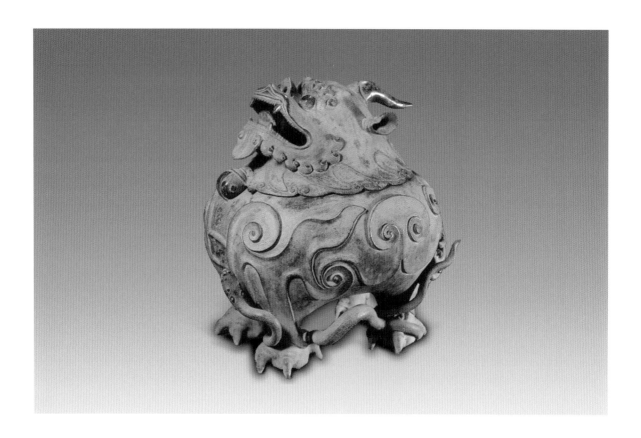

兽形铜熏炉

明

铜质

口径 17 厘米，通高 33 厘米

Bronze Beast-shaped Incense Burner

Ming Dynasty

Bronze

Mouth Diameter 17 cm/ Height 33 cm

炉呈独角怪兽形，昂首挺立，利齿交错。腹部饰卷云纹，尾部分开均向内卷，足部有一缠绕四足的蛇，兽首为熏炉盖，腹内中空，嘴、眼、耳通透，以散发香味。

河北博物院藏

The whole incense burner resembles a unicorn that stands firmly with the raised head and sharp and interlacing teeth. Its belly is decorated with curly cloud patterns. There is a snake twining around the four paws of the beast. The head of the unicorn is the lid of the burner. Its belly has a hollow space that is connected with its mouth, eyes and ears for emitting fragrance.

Preserved in Hebei Museum

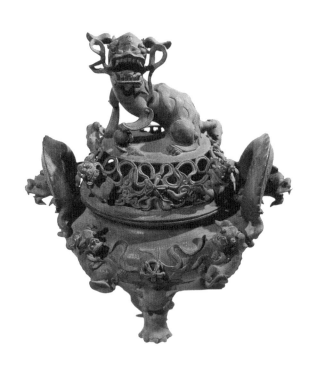

麒麟熏炉

明

铜质

口径 28 厘米，高 50 厘米

Incense Burner with Kylin Designs

Ming Dynasty

Bronze

Diameter 28 cm/ Height 50 cm

炉上部为盖，透雕云纹，有 4 只麒麟，顶部
饰一只大麒麟，瞠目露齿。下部为炉体，侈
口，鼓腹，三兽蹄足，双立耳，器表浮雕纹饰。
为室内香熏器。

上海中医药博物馆藏

The lid of the burner is furnished with openwork
carvings of cloud patterns and four kylins. A
big kylin is standing on the lid with its eyes and
mouth wide open. The burner has a wide flared
mouth, a bulged belly, three paw-shaped feet,
and two erect handles. The surface of the burner
is decorated with patterns in relief. The burner
was used for indoor aromatherapy.

Preserved in Shanghai Museum of Traditional
Chinese Medicine

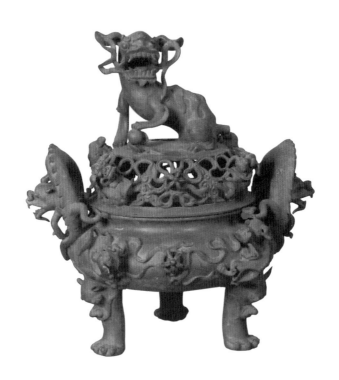

麒麟熏炉

明

铜质

宽 46 厘米，通高 51 厘米

Incense Burner with Kylin Designs

Ming Dynasty

Bronze

Width 46 cm/ Height 51 cm

炉上部为盖，镂空，盖顶伏麒麟钮。下部为
炉体，侈口，鼓腹，三兽蹄足，双立耳，耳
上饰兽头，器表浮雕纹饰。1974 年入藏。

中华医学会 / 上海中医药大学医史博物馆藏

The upper part of the burner is a pierced cover
decorated with openwork patterns. A kylin,
standing on the top of the cover, serves as the
knob. The lower part is the body of the burner
which has a wide flared mouth, a bulged belly,
three paw-shaped feet, and two erect handles
with beast-head designs. The surface of the
burner is decorated with patterns in relief. The
incense burner was collected in 1974.

Preserved in Chinese Medical Association/
Museum of Chinese Medicine, Shanghai
University of Traditional Chinese Medicine

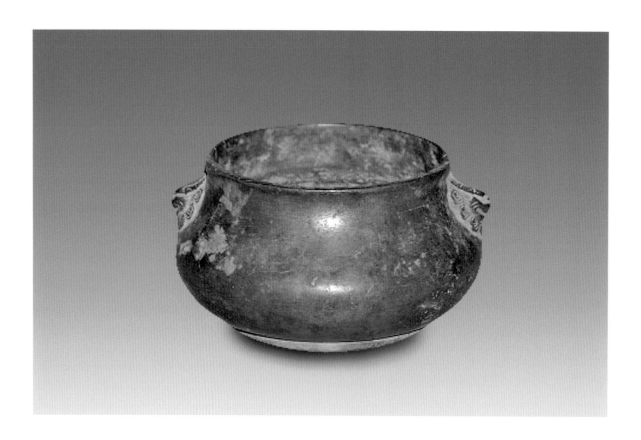

宣德款铜炉

明

铜质

口径 9 厘米，底径 7.8 厘米，通高 6 厘米，重 400 克

Bronze Incense Burner of Xuande Period

Ming Dynasty

Bronze

Mouth Diameter 9 cm/ Bottom Diameter 7.8 cm/ Height 6 cm/ Weight 400 g

侈口，扁腹，圈足，两兽耳。底有铭文"大
明宣德年制"，腹部有一小孔。为礼器。陕
西省咸阳市秦都区征集。

陕西医史博物馆藏

This incense burner has a wide flared mouth, a
flat and round belly, a ring foot, and two beast-
shaped handles. The Chinese characters "Da
Ming Xuan De Nian Zhi" on the bottom mean
that the burner was made during Xuande Period
of the Ming Dynasty. The burner served as a
sacrificial vessel. It was collected in Qindu
District of Xianyang City, Shaanxi Province.
Preserved in Shaanxi Museum of Medical History

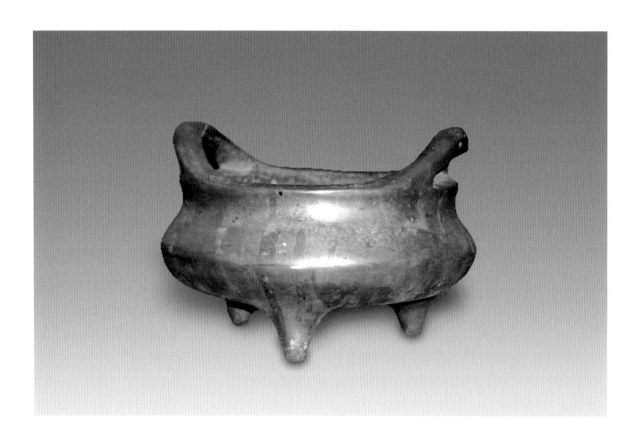

宣德款铜炉

明

铜质

口径 21.5 厘米，底径 21 厘米，通高 15 厘米，重 5150 克

Bronze Incense Burner of Xuande Period

Ming Dynasty

Bronze

Mouth Diameter 21.5 cm/ Bottom Diameter 21 cm/ Height 15 cm/ Weight 5,150 g

直口，口沿上带双耳，折腹，乳状足。底有"大明宣德制"的字样。为礼器、生活用器。

陕西医史博物馆藏

This incense burner has a vertical mouth, a flat and bulged belly, a ring base, and two handles on the rim of the mouth. The six characters "Da Ming Xuan De Nian Zhi" on the bottom mean that the burner was made during Xuande Period of the Ming Dynasty. The incense burner served as a sacrificial vessel and daily household utensil. Preserved in Shaanxi Museum of Medical History

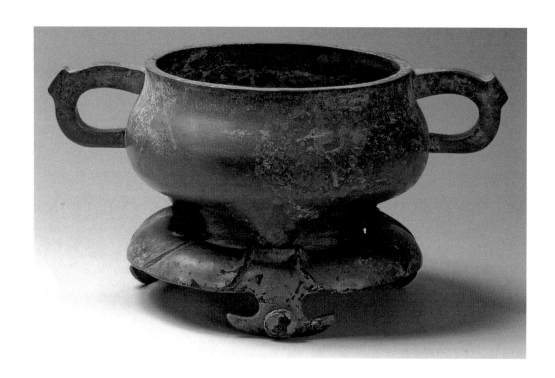

宣德款铜炉

明

铜质

高 16.2 厘米

Bronze Incense Burner of Xuande Period

Ming Dynasty

Bronze

Height 16.2 cm

直口，鼓腹内收，平底，下承三足，双竖耳。

底部铸"大明宣德年制"款铭。通体造型简朴，

包浆光润。传南京南郊出土。

南京市博物馆藏

This incense burner has a vertical mouth, a
bulged belly, a flat bottom, three feet, and two
erect handles. The six characters "Da Ming
Xuan De Nian Zhi" on the bottom mean that the
burner was made during Xuande Period of the
Ming Dynasty. The design of the burner with
smooth wrapped slurry is simple. It is said the
burner was unearthed on the southern suburbs
of Nanjing City.

Preserved in Nanjing Municipal Museum

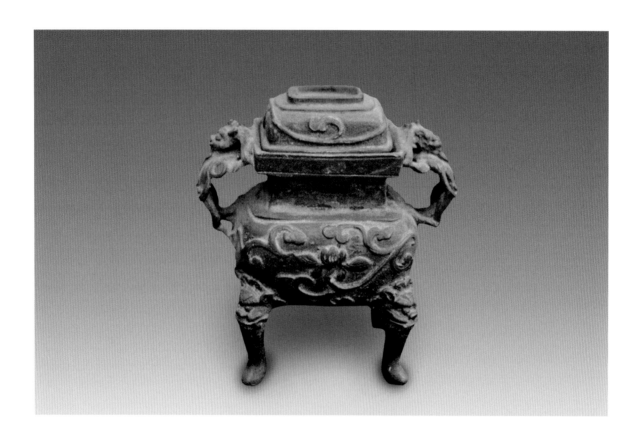

堆花铜香炉

明

铜质

长 8.1 厘米，宽 5.2 厘米，通高 8.8 厘米，腹深 5.3 厘米，重 250 克

Bronze Incense Burner with Flower Designs

Ming Dynasty

Bronze

Length 8.1 cm/ Width 5.2 cm/ Height 8.8 cm/ Belly Depth 5.3 cm/ Weight 250 g

形似鼎，方形直口，方圆形鼓腹，四兽蹄形足，兽形双耳，有方形盖。器表堆花纹饰。

广东中医药博物馆藏

The incense burner resembles a ding vessel, with a square and vertical mouth. It has a square and round belly, four paw-shaped feet, two beast-shaped handles, and a square lid. Its surface is decorated with flowers in stacks.

Preserved in Guangdong Chinese Medicine Museum

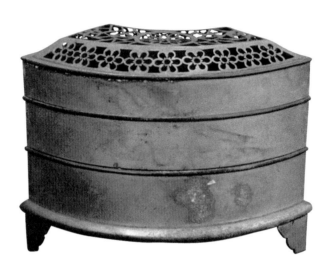

铜熏香扇形炉

明

铜质

外围周长 12.5 厘米，内围周长 5.4 厘米，宽 5.1 厘米，通高 9 厘米，重 238 克

Bronze Sector-shaped Incense Burner

Ming Dynasty

Bronze

Outer Circumference 12.5 cm/ Inner Circumference 5.4 cm/ Width 5.1 cm/ Height 9 cm/ Weight 238 g

扇形，上面镂空，直腹，扁平足。炉内放燃
香料，香味由镂空面飘散出去。

广东中医药博物馆藏

The incense burner is in the shape of a sector,
with a hollowed-out top, a vertical belly, and
flat feet. When incense was placed in the burner,
the fragrance came out from its pierced top.
Preserved in Guangdong Chinese Medicine
Museum

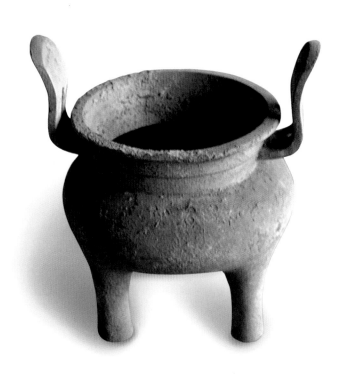

鼎

明

铜质

口径 14.5 厘米，高 17 厘米

Ding Vessel

Ming Dynasty

Bronze

Mouth Diameter 14.5 cm/ Height 17 cm

侈口，鼓腹，三圆柱形足，双立耳。为礼器、炊器。由成都市博物馆调拨。

成都中医药大学中医药传统文化博物馆藏

The vessel has a wide flared mouth, a bulged belly, three cylindrical feet, and two erect handles. It was an ancient sacrificial and cooking vessel. It was allocated from Chengdu Museum

Preserved in Museum of Traditional Chinese Medicine Culture, Chengdu University of Traditional Chinese Medicine

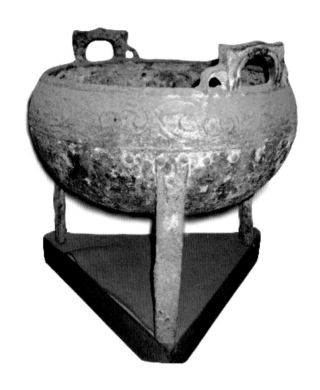

铁鼎

明

铁质

口径 61 厘米，通高 62.5 厘米，足高 39 厘米

Iron Ding Vessel

Ming Dynasty

Iron

Mouth Diameter 61 cm/ Height 62.5 cm/ Foot Height 39 cm

敛口，鼓腹，双耳立于口沿，三锥状足，腹
上有浮雕。为礼器、炊器。陕西省澄城县冯
原乡征集。

陕西医史博物馆藏

The vessel has a contracted mouth, a bulged
belly, three conical feet, and two erect handles
on the rim of the mouth. Its belly is embossed
with patterns. The vessel was an ancient
sacrificial and cooking vessel. It was collected
from Fengyuan of Chengcheng County, Shaanxi
Province.

Preserved in Shaanxi Museum of Medical History

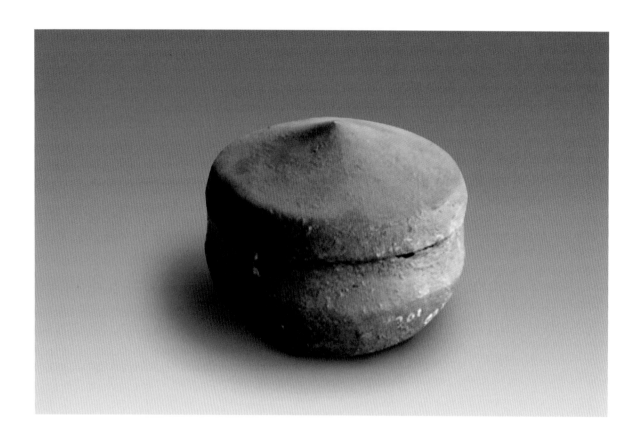

盒

明

铁质

口径 11.5 厘米，高 7 厘米

Box

Ming Dynasty

Iron

Mouth Diameter 11.5 cm/ Height 7 cm

鼓腹，平底，盖中部为尖状，腹部稍残。由
成都市考古队调拨。

　　成都中医药大学中医药传统文化博物馆藏

The box has a bulged belly, a flat bottom and
a pointed lid. The belly is slightly damaged. It
was allocated from Chengdu Archaeological
Team.

Preserved in Museum of Traditional Chinese
Medicine Culture, Chengdu University of
Traditional Chinese Medicine

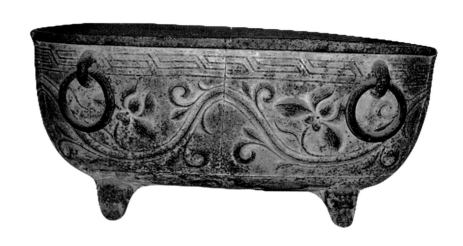

铁盒

明

铁质

长口径 104 厘米，宽 57.6 厘米，通高 44 厘米

Iron Box

Ming Dynasty

Iron

Maximum Mouth Diameter 104 cm/ Width 57.6 cm/ Height 44 cm

长方形口，直腹，四兽足。沿下垂环，现缺
一只环，腹上有浮雕莲花纹。为生活器具。
陕西省鄠邑区征集。

陕西医史博物馆收藏

The box has an oblong mouth, a vertical belly,
four paw-shaped feet, and four drooping rings
with one missing. Its belly is embossed with
lotus flowers. The box was collected in Huyi
District, Shaanxi Province.

Preserved in Shaanxi Museum of Medical History

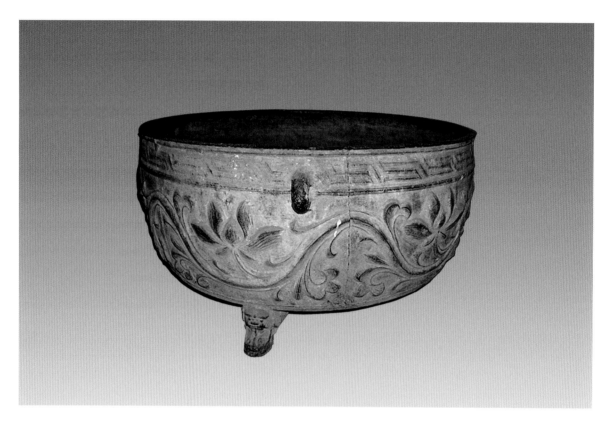

铁盒

明

铁质

长口径 111 厘米，短口径 63 厘米，通高 49.4 厘米

Iron Box

Ming Dynasty

Iron

Maximum Mouth Diameter 111 cm/ Width 63 cm/ Height 49.4 cm

椭圆形口，圈底，四兽足。沿下四环，现缺三
只环，腹上有浮雕莲花纹。为生活器具。陕西
省鄠邑区征集。

陕西医史博物馆收藏

The box has an oblong mouth, a vertical belly,
four paw-shaped feet, and four lugs below the rim
with three ones missing. The belly is embossed
with lotus flowers. The box was a daily appliance. It
was collected in Huyi Distrid, Shaanxi Province.
Preserved in Shaanxi Museum of Medical History

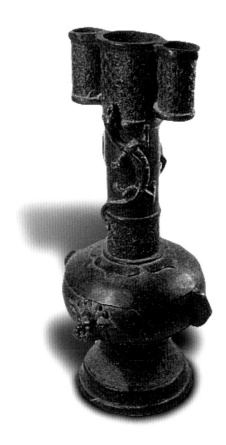

铁投壶

明

铁质

口径 3.6 厘米，高 26 厘米，耳径 2.3 厘米，耳
长 4.2 厘米

Iron Pitch-pot

Ming Dynasty

Iron

Mouth Diameter 3.6 cm/ Height 26 cm/ Handle

Diameter 2.3 cm/ Handle Length 4.2 cm

长颈，附双坚耳，鼓腹，圜底，圈足。绕颈部铸有一龙，腹部分铸有四只兽头。此壶的造型与宋司马光《投壶新格》中有关投壶形制的描述完全一致，为宋元以来投壶的基本样式。

中国体育博物馆藏

The pitch-pot has a long neck, two solid ears, a bulged belly, a round bottom, and a ring foot. A dragon surrounds the pot's neck. Four beast heads are cast on the belly. The pitch-pot was patterned exactly the same as the one depicted in *New Etiquettes for Playing Pitch-pots* written by Sima Guang of the Song Dynasty. This was a very classic pitch-pot during the Song Dynasty and the Yuan Dynasty.

Preserved in China Sports Museum

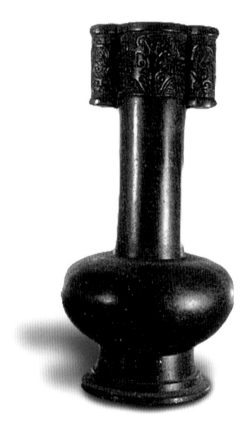

铜投壶

明

铜质

口径 3.4 厘米，高 18.9 厘米，耳径 1.4 厘米

Bronze Pitch-pot

Ming Dynasty

Bronze

Mouth Diameter 3.4 cm/ Height 18.9 cm/ Handle
Diameter 1.4 cm

长颈，鼓腹，下附圜底，圈足，口部附有双坚耳，表面皆铸有兽面纹。此为一种小型投壶。

中国体育博物馆藏

The pitch-pot, which is of small type, has a long neck, a bulged belly, and a round bottom with a ring foot. There is one solid ear at each side of the mouth. The surface is decorated with beast's face patterns.

Preserved in China Sports Museum

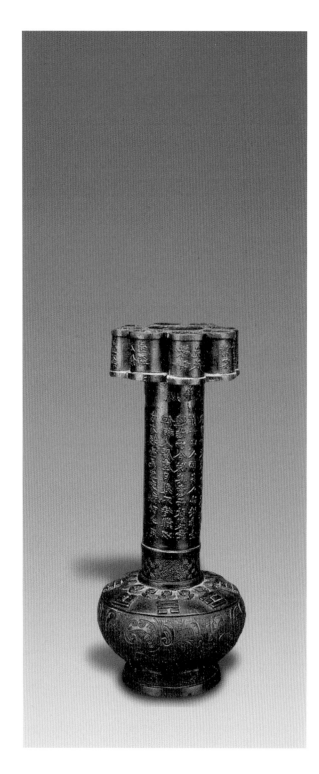

铜投壶

明

铜质

通高 35 厘米

Bronze Pitch-pot

Ming Dynasty

Bronze

Height 35 cm

长颈，下鼓腹，附以圜底，圈足。口部附有 8 个小竖耳。竖耳和壶的颈部皆铸有文字，腹部和图足铸有兽面纹。此为明代投壶活动中较为常用的一种投壶造型。

法国吉美国立亚洲艺术博物馆藏

The pitch-pot has a long neck, eight lugs, a bulged belly, and a round bottom with a ring foot. Its lugs and neck are decorated with Chinese characters while its belly and base are patterned with beast's faces. This was a very classic type of pitch-pots in the Ming Dynasty.

Preserved in Musée National des Arts Asiatiques-Guimet, France

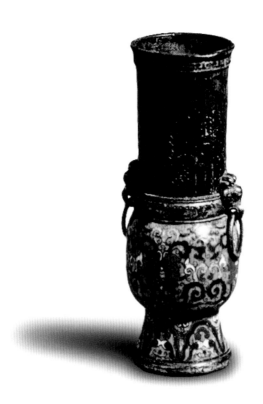

珐琅彩铜投壶

明

铜质

口径 12 厘米，高 26 厘米

Enamel Pitch-pot

Ming Dynasty

Bronze

Mouth Diameter 12 cm/ Height 26 cm

颈部修长，直口，鼓腹，底附圈足，颈腹之
间有两环耳，外表皆饰以珐琅彩。此为投壶
中的一种独特样式。

中国体育博物馆藏

The pitch-pot has a slender neck, a vertical
mouth, a bulged belly, a ring base, and two
ring handles between the neck and the belly. Its
surface is decorated with enamel designs, which
makes it a very special type of pitch-pot.

Preserved in China Sports Museum

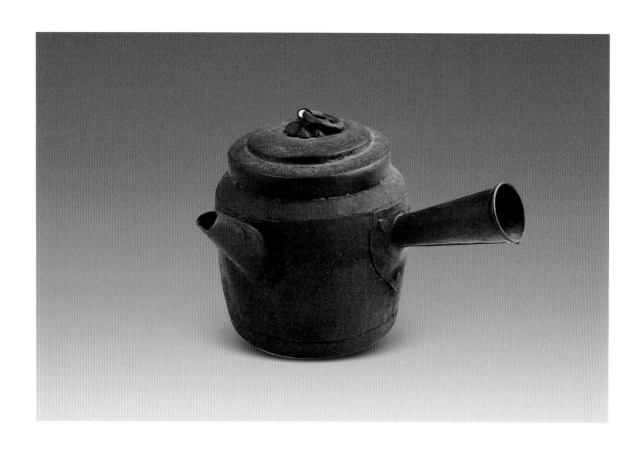

熬药壶

明

金属质

高 24 厘米，口径 16 厘米，壶把长 10 厘米，壶嘴 6 厘米

Medicine-decocting Pot

Ming Dynasty

Metal

Height 24 cm/ Mouth Diameter 16 cm/ Length of Handle 10 cm/ Mouth of Handle 6 cm

直口，平沿，溜肩，直腹，腹上铸流，直把，把与腹遁形连接，有三铆钉，配盖。明代熬制中药的器皿。

北京御生堂中医药博物馆藏

The pot has a vertical mouth, a flat edge, an inclined shoulder, a spout, and a lid. A vertical handle is connected with the belly with three rivets. The pot was used for decocting medicine in the Qing Dynasty.
Preserved in Chinese Medicine Museum of Beijing Yu Sheng Tang Drugstore

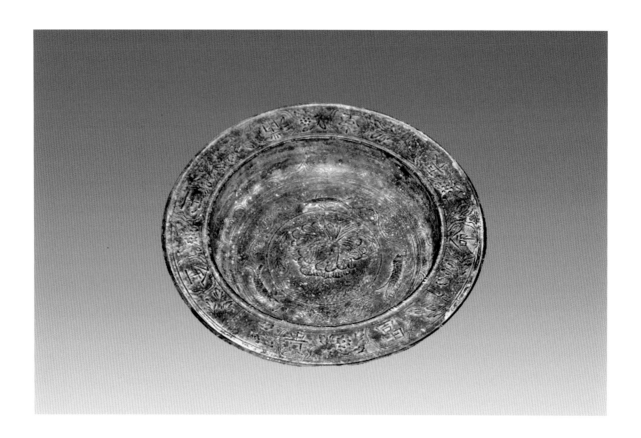

铜盘

明

铜质

口径 30.2 厘米，底径 20 厘米，通高 6 厘米，重 2450 克

Bronze Basin

Ming Dynasty

Bronze

Mouth Diameter 30.2 cm/ Bottom Diameter 20 cm/ Height 6 cm/ Weight 2,450 g

平沿，三足。沿上有"富贵满堂，金玉常命"
的字样，盘内底雕有荷花图。为生活器具。
陕西省咸阳市博物馆调拨，1978 年入藏。

陕西医史博物馆藏

The basin has a flat rim and three feet. The
orifice is decorated with Chinese characters
"Fu Gui Man Tang, Jin Yu Chang Ming",
which means wealth, longevity and prosperity
of the family. The inner bottom of the basin is
patterned with a lotus. It was an item for daily
use. It was collected from Xianyang Museum,
in 1978.

Preserved in Shaanxi Museum of Medical History

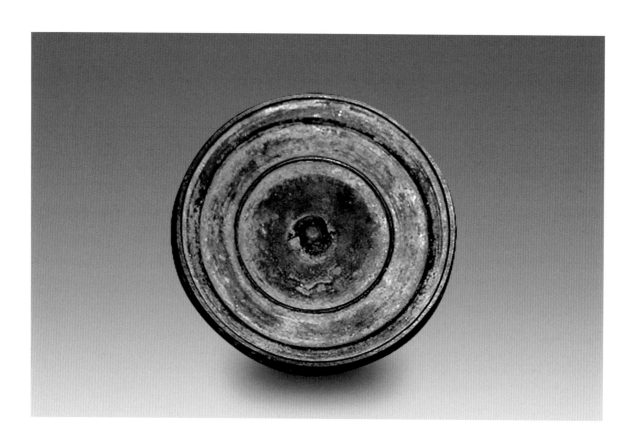

铜镜

明

铜质

直径 8 厘米，重 150 克

圆形，圆钮。边沿为凸棱，无纹饰。为生活器具。

陕西医史博物馆藏

Bronze Mirror

Ming Dynasty

Bronze

Diameter 8 cm/ Weight 150 g

The plain mirror is circular in shape with a hemispherical knob. Its edge is raised. The mirror was an item for daily use.

Preserved in Shaanxi Museum of Medical History

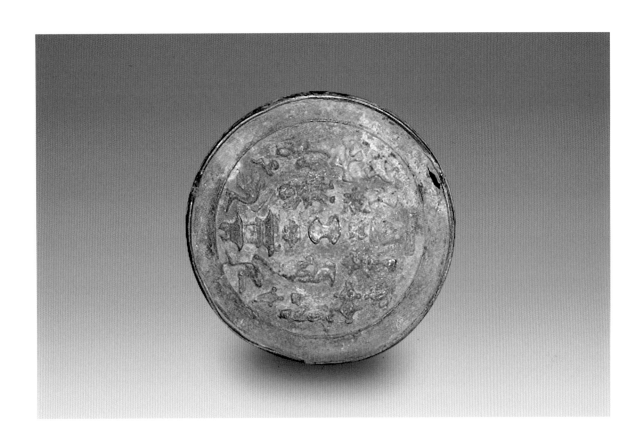

铜镜

明

铜质

直径 12.8 厘米，高 0.4 厘米，重 250 克

圆形，桥形钮。内区饰人物飞禽图案。为生活用器。陕西历史博物馆调拨。

陕西医史博物馆藏

Bronze Mirror

Ming Dynasty

Bronze

Diameter 12.8 cm/ Height 0.4 cm/ Weight 250 g

The mirror is circular in shape with a bridge-shaped knob. Its inner segment is decorated with patterns of figures and birds. The mirror was an item for daily use. It was allocated from Shaanxi History Museum.

Preserved in Shaanxi Museum of Medical History

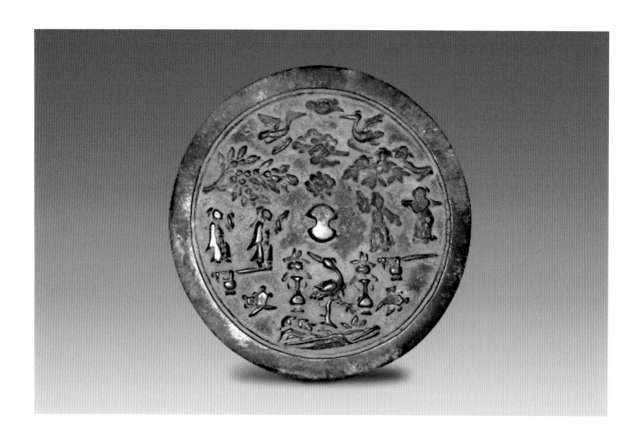

铜镜

明

铜质

直径 15 厘米，高 0.4 厘米，镜边沿宽 1.5 厘米，重 500 克

Bronze Mirror

Ming Dynasty

Bronze

Diameter 15 cm/ Height 0.4 cm/ Rim Width 1.5 cm/ Weight 500 g

圆形。桥形钮。内区饰人物飞禽图案。为生
活用具。陕西省咸阳市征集。

陕西医史博物馆藏

The mirror is circular in shape with a bridge-
shaped knob. Its inner region is decorated with
patterns of figures and birds. It was an item for
daily use. The mirror was collected in Xianyang
City, Shaanxi Province.

Preserved in Shaanxi Museum of Medical
History

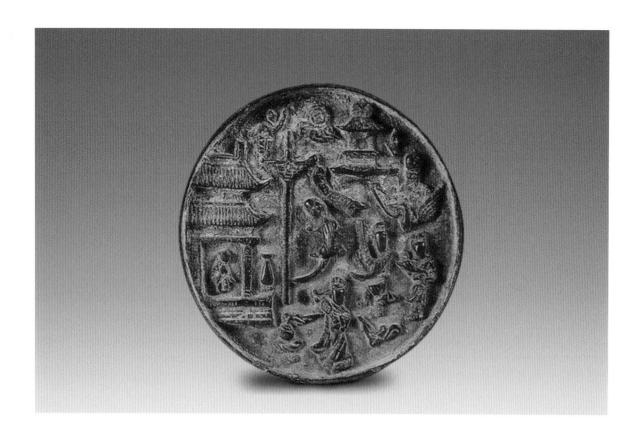

技巧纹铜镜

明

铜质

直径 10.2 厘米

Bronze Mirror with Acrobatic Scene

Ming Dynasty

Bronze

Diameter 10.2 cm

圆形。无钮。整个铜镜纹饰描绘的是一幅乐舞图案，图案中部一竖起的横竿上，一伎人张开双臂站立于顶部的横杆上,做表演动作。周围有乐队伴奏。画面简朴，技巧动作设计颇具特色。1957年河北省巨鹿县出土。

The mirror is round in shape without a knob. The back of the mirror is decorated with a scene of acrobatic performance. In the middle part there is an erect pole, on the top of which stands a man performing with a music band playing around. The picture is simple and plain with a unique feature. The mirror was unearthed in Julu County, Hebei Province, in 1957.

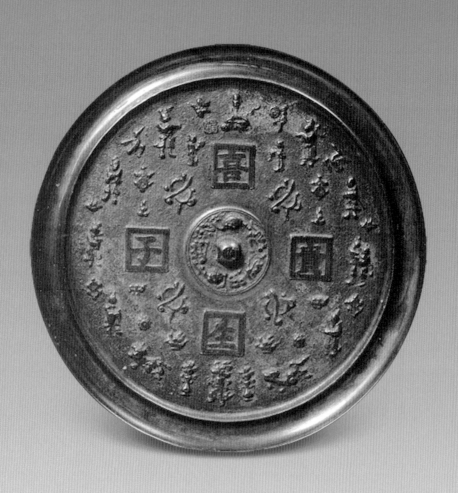

喜生贵子铜镜

明

铜质

直径 35 厘米

圆形。银锭式钮，圆形钮座上有浮雕纹饰。有"喜生贵子"吉祥铭文，纹样为传统题材，有龙凤鱼虫，人物故事，吉祥八宝等。传出土于南京。

南京市博物馆藏

Bronze Mirror Patterned with Congratulations on Birth

Ming Dynasty

Bronze

Diameter 35 cm

The mirror is round with an ingot-shaped knob on the embossed hemispherical base. The middle part of the mirror is decorated with traditional auspicious patterns including phoenixes, dragons, figures and Chinese characters "Xi Sheng Gui Zi", which means congratulations on the birth of a son. It is said the mirror was unearthed on Nanjing City.

Preserved in Nanjing Municipal Museum

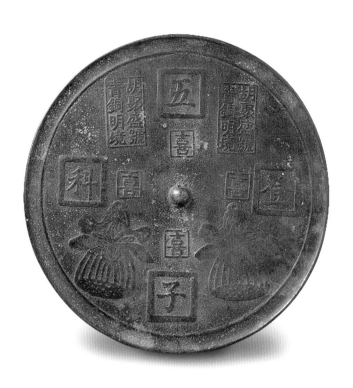

五子登科镜

明

铜质

直径 20.7 厘米

Mirror with Designs of Passing Imperial Examination

Ming Dynasty

Bronze

Diameter 20.7 cm

圆形。圆钮。镜背素地，饰"五子登科"四字，每字内侧对应一"喜"字，每字均用方栏圈起。"五"字两侧长方栏内铸"胡聚盛号青铜明镜"八字，"子"字两侧饰以莲蓬纹，取"连生贵子"之意。五子登科是当时常用的吉语。

中国国家博物馆藏

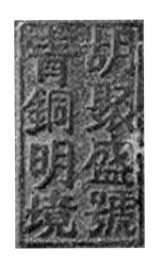

The mirror is circular in shape with a hemispherical knob. Its back is decorated with Chinese characters, among which the four in the big squares "Wu Zi Deng Ke" mean passing the imperial examination; the four in the small squares " 喜 "mean happiness; the ones in the oblong squares are the name of the workshop where the mirror was made. At the bottom of the mirror there is a lotus seedpod on each side of the character " 子 " (son), implying successive birth of sons. "Wu Zi Dong Ke" is the auspicious language commonly used in that times.

Preserved in National Museum of China

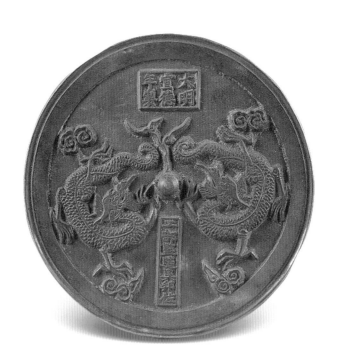

宣德吴邦佐造双龙镜

明

铜质

直径 21 厘米

Mirror with the Design of Two Dragons

Ming Dynasty

Bronze

Diameter 21 cm

圆形。圆钮。内区双龙夹钮对峙，口对钮珠，昂首盘曲。隙间饰四朵祥云。钮上方有铭文"大明宣德年制"六字，钮下长方栏内有铭文"工部监造吴邦佐"七字。双重三角缘。镜体厚重，制作规整。

中国国家博物馆藏

The mirror is circular in shape with a hemispherical knob. In the inner segment there are two coiled dragons facing each other with their heads raised toward the knob. The interstice is decorated with four auspicious clouds. Above the knob there are six Chinese characters indicating the year when the mirror was made. In the oblong column beneath the knob there are seven inscriptions of the supervisor's name. The mirror, which is thick and heavy, has double triangular rims.

Preserved in National Museum of China

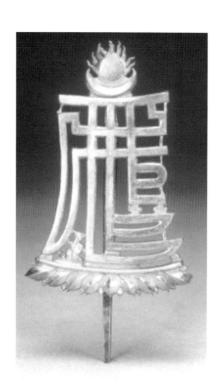

梵文金发簪

明

金质

宽 5.8 厘米，通长 12 厘米，重 31 克

Gold Hairpin with Sanskrit Characters

Ming Dynasty

Gold

Width 5.8 cm/ Length 12 cm/ Weight 31 g

簪首用薄金片制成，上端为日月、火焰图案，中间为一镂空梵文，下以连珠纹和莲花瓣作边饰。簪卡身为银质，固定于簪首背面。这件发簪具有浓郁的宗教色彩。

常州博物馆藏

The face of the hairpin is made of a gold sheet decorated with patterns of the moon, the sun and flames on the top, pierced Sanskrit characters in the middle, a string of pearls at the bottom, and lotus petals at the edge. Its pin is made of silver. This hairpin has a strong religious feature.

Preserved in Changzhou Museum

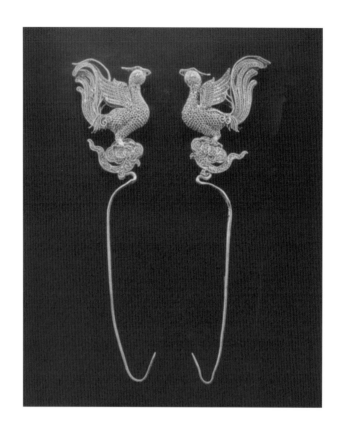

垒丝金凤装饰

明

金质

长 22.3 厘米

Gold Accessories for Phoenix Coronet

Ming Dynasty

Gold

Length 22.3 cm

此系凤冠上的插饰。凤首与凤爪用叠珠方法
垒成，凤尾、凤翅均垒编制成；羽毛部分则
采用将两股金丝缠绕后再垒叠的方法。多种
工艺，分段制作，最后焊接合成，技术十分
精湛，代表了明代金银细工的高超水平。南
京太平门外徐达家族墓出土。

南京市博物馆藏

These exquisite artifacts are the accessories
for a phoenix coronet. They were made with
many techniques including stacking, weaving,
twining, filigreeing and welding. The exquisite
workmanship represented the high level of gold
and silver ware making in the Ming and Qing
Dynasties. The collection was unearthed from
the family tomb of Xu Da in Nanjing City.
Preserved in Nanjing Municipal Museum

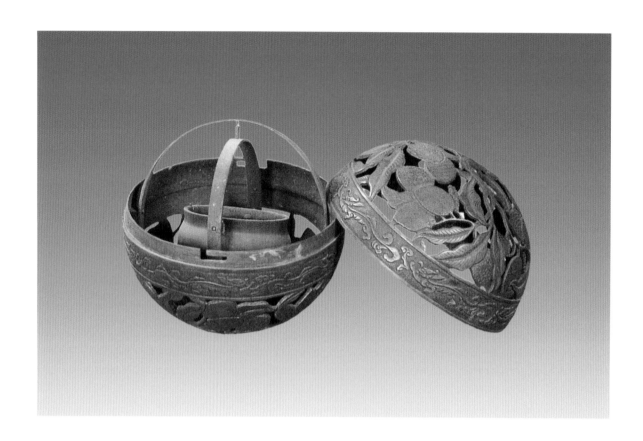

透雕镂空床熏

明

铜质

腹径 12.8 厘米，高 12 厘米

Hollowed-out Incense Burner for Bedding

Ming Dynasty

Bronze

Belly Diameter 12.8 cm/ Height 12 cm

圆球形，全镂空。分上下两半，内部有两个
同心机环，机环有轴承，环内有盂。熏球转
动时，香盂始终保持平衡，可香熏消毒被褥
用，故亦名"卧褥香炉"。

上海中医药博物馆藏

This incense burner is in the shape of a ball
and is hollow inside. There is a container for
the incense in the ball which balances well
when the ball is rolling. It was used for disinfecting
bedding. It also named as "Wo Chuang Xiang Lu".
Preserved in Shanghai Museum of Traditional
Chinese

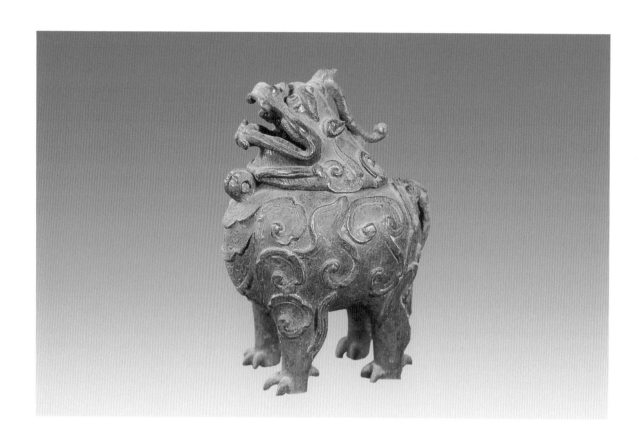

帽熏

明

铜质

长 11 厘米，宽 10 厘米，高 18 厘米

Incense Burner for Caps

Ming Dynasty

Bronze

Length 11 cm/ Width 10 cm/ Height 18 cm

獬豸形，昂首挺立。腹部饰卷云纹，尾下垂，

四足带爪，腹内中空。用于香熏消毒帽子。

上海中医药博物馆藏

The whole incense burner resembles a haetae,
a legendary mythical creature. The belly of
incense burner is patterned with cirrus cloud
designs. It is standing erectly with a drooping
tail and four paws. Its belly is a container for incense.
The burner was used for disinfecting caps.
Preserved in Shanghai Museum of Traditional
Chinese Medicine

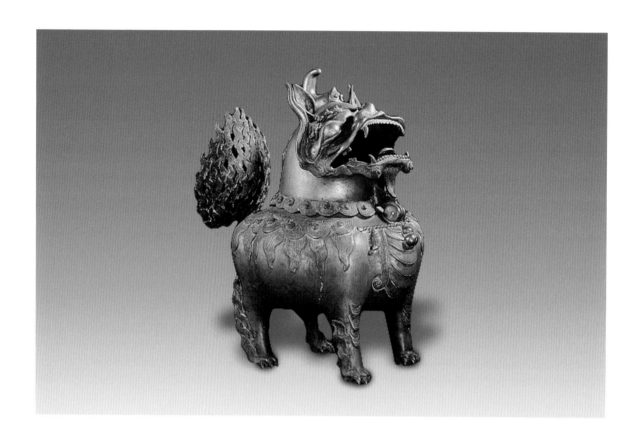

獬豸熏

明

铜质

长 47 厘米，宽 34 厘米，高 57 厘米

Haetae-shaped Incense Burner

Ming Dynasty

Bronze

Length 47 cm/ Width 34 cm/ Height 57 cm

獬豸形，为传说中的公正严明的祥兽。昂首瞪眼挺立，颈肩部有鬃毛，尾上翘，四足带爪，腹内中空。头部可掀开，内放置点燃香料药物，香熏室内之用。

上海中医药博物馆藏

The whole incense burner resembles a haetae, a legendary mythical creature. It is standing erectly with its head raised and its eyes glaring. Its neck and shoulders are covered with mane and its tail curls upwards. It has four paws. Its head is the lid of the incense burner. The body has a hollow space as a container for spices and medicinal herbs. The device was used for indoor aromatherapy.

Preserved in Shanghai Museum of Traditional Chinese Medicine

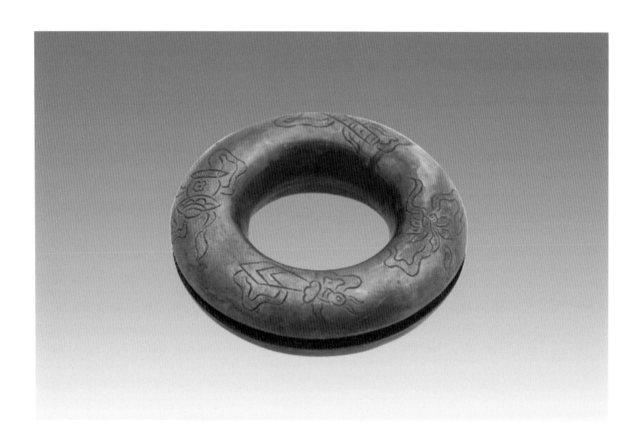

串铃

明

铜质

直径 16 厘米

Bell

Ming Dynasty

Bronze

Diameter 16 cm

半封闭环状铜圈，雕刻精美花纹。又名"虎撑"或"虎衔"，行医卖药者外出时必备之物，后人逐渐将铜圈改成手摇的响器。行医标志，表示自己是能医龙治虎的药王弟子；二来是因为孙思邈用这只铜圈救了老虎而没被吃掉，郎中便把它作为保护自己行医的护身符了。医生使用串铃也有很多讲究。一是使用者根据自己医术的高明程度使用大小不同，医术高的一般用稍大一些的。还有就是使用时，初学者摇串铃不能超过胸口，中级水平者不能超过肩头，只有高水平医生才能举过头顶摇，所以当时在中医行业内部已经有相对完善的自律与监督。

北京御生堂中医药博物馆藏

The half-closed circular bronze ring, also known as Hu Cheng and Hu Xian, is carved with exquisite patterns. It was the gadget of medical practitioners or medicine sellers when they went out for practice or business. People in later time gradually changed the bronze ring into a hand-shaken percussion gadget. It is a medical practitioner' symbol which implies he was a disciple of the King of Medicine, who could treat dragons' or tigers' diseases. It was also used by medical practitioners as their amulet because Sun Simiao, the King of Medicine, used this bronze ring to save a tiger without being killed. The usage of different size of bells depends on the varied degree of practitioners' medical skills. A skillful practitioner could use a bigger one. A beginner should shake it below his chest. A practitioner of intermediate level could not shake it above his shoulder while only a senior one could shake it over his head, which showed sound self-discipline and supervision in the industry of traditional Chinese medicine.

Preserved in Chinese Medicine Museum of Beijing Yu Sheng Tang Drugstore

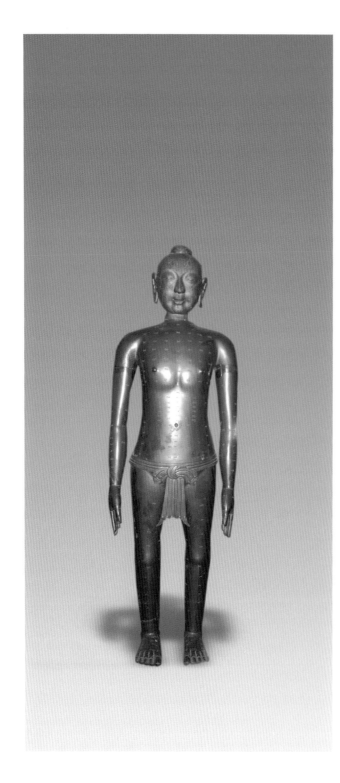

仿宋铜人

明

铜质

高 18.6 厘米

Copper Man Model Simulated from Song Dynasty

Ming Dynasty

Plaster

Height 18.6 cm

为一成年男子正面站立形象，体表标明针灸腧穴、穴名及经络循行等。教学模具。20 世纪70 年代入藏，中国国家博物馆复制。完整无损。

陕西医史博物馆藏

The statue is a man standing facing front. The body surface is marked with the positions of acupuncture and moxibustion points, the names of the acupoints and the flow of the main and collateral channels. It was utilized as teaching aids. It was collected in the 1970s and is a duplicate from National Museum of China. It is still in good condition.

Preserved in Shaanxi Museum of Medicine History

索　引

Index

534

参考文献

[1] 李经纬.中国古代医史图录[M].北京：人民卫生出版社，1992.

[2] 傅维康，李经纬，林昭庚.中国医学通史：文物图谱卷[M].北京：人民卫生出版社，2000.

[3] 和中浚，吴鸿洲.中华医学文物图集[M].成都：四川人民出版社，2001.

[4] 上海中医药博物馆.上海中医药博物馆馆藏珍品[M].上海：上海科学技术出版社，2013.

[5] 西藏自治区博物馆.西藏博物馆[M].北京：五洲传播出版社，2005.

[6] 崔乐泉.中国古代体育文物图录：中英文本[M].北京：中华书局，2000.

[7] 张金明，陆雪春.中国古铜镜鉴赏图录[M].北京：中国民族摄影艺术出版社，2002.

[8] 文物精华编辑委会员.文物精华[M].北京：文物出版社，1964.

[9] 谭维四.湖北出土文物精华[M].武汉：湖北教育出版社，2001.

[10] 常州市博物馆.常州文物精华[M].北京：文物出版社，1998.

[11] 镇江博物馆.镇江文物精华[M].合肥：黄山书社，1997.

[12] 贵州省文化厅，贵州省博物馆.贵州文物精华[M].贵阳：贵州人民出版社，2005.

[13] 徐良玉.扬州馆藏文物精华[M].南京：江苏古籍出版社，2001.

[14] 昭陵博物馆，陕西历史博物馆.昭陵文物精华[M].西安：陕西人民美术出版社，1991.

[15] 南通博物苑.南通博物苑文物精华[M].北京：文物出版社，2005.

[16] 邯郸市文物研究所.邯郸文物精华[M].北京：文物出版社，2005.

[17] 张秀生，刘友恒，聂连顺，等.中国河北正定文物精华[M].北京：文化艺术出版社，1998.

[18] 陕西省咸阳市文物局.咸阳文物精华[M].北京：文物出版社，2002.

[19] 安阳市文物管理局.安阳文物精华[M].北京：文物出版社，2004.

[20] 深圳市博物馆.深圳市博物馆文物精华[M].北京：文物出版社，1998.

[21]《中国文物精华》编辑委员会.中国文物精华（1993）[M].北京：文物出版社，1993.

[22] 夏路，刘永生.山西省博物馆馆藏文物精华 [M].太原：山西人民出版社，1999.

[23] 文物精华编辑委员会.文物精华 [M].文物出版社，1957.

[24] 山西博物院，湖北省博物馆.荆楚长歌：九连墩楚墓出土文物精华 [M].太原：山西人民出版社，2011.

[25] 刘广堂，石金鸣，宋建忠.晋国雄风：山西出土两周文物精华 [M].沈阳：万卷出版公司，2009.

[26] 沈君山，王国平，单迎红.滦平博物馆馆藏文物精华 [M].北京：中国文联出版社，2012.

[27] 张家口市博物馆.张家口市博物馆馆藏文物精华 [M].北京：科学出版社，2011.

[28] 浙江省文物考古研究所.浙江考古精华 [M].北京：文物出版社，1999.

[29] 故宫博物院.故宫雕刻珍萃 [M].北京：紫禁城出版社，2004.

[30] 故宫博物院紫禁城出版社.故宫博物院藏宝录 [M].上海：上海文艺出版社，1986.

[31] 首都博物馆.大元三都 [M].北京：科学出版社，2016.

[32] 新疆维吾尔自治区博物馆.新疆出土文物 [M].北京：文物出版社，1975.

[33] 王兴伊，段逸山.新疆出土涉医文书辑校 [M].上海：上海科学技术出版社，2016.

[34] 刘学春.刍议医药卫生文物的概念与分类标准 [J].中华中医药杂志，2016，31（11）:4406-4409.

[35] 上海古籍出版社.中国艺海 [M].上海：上海古籍出版社，1994.

[36] 紫都，岳鑫.一生必知的 200 件国宝 [M].呼和浩特：远方出版社，2005.

[37] 谭维四.湖北出土文物精华 [M].武汉：湖北教育出版社，2001.

[38] 张建青.青海彩陶收藏与鉴赏 [M].北京：中国文史出版社，2007.

[39] 银景琦.仡佬族文物 [M].南宁：广西人民出版社，2014.

[40] 廖果，梁峻，李经纬.东西方医学的反思与前瞻 [M].北京：中医古籍出版社，2002.

[41] 梁峻，张志斌，廖果，等.中华医药文明史集论 [M].北京：中医古籍出版社，2003.

[42] 郑蓉，庄乾竹，刘聪，等.中国医药文化遗产考论 [M].北京：中医古籍出版社，2005.